Emergencies in Otorhinolaryngology

Emergencies in Otorhinolaryngology

GC Sahoo
Retd Professor and Head
Department of ENT
Rajah Muthiah Medical College and Hospital
Annamalai University
Annamalai Nagar, Tamil Nadu, India

Forewords

Abhoya Kumar Kar
Rankanidhi Samal

JAYPEE

JAYPEE BROTHERS MEDICAL PUBLISHERS
The Health Sciences Publisher
New Delhi | London

JAYPEE **Jaypee Brothers Medical Publishers (P) Ltd**

Headquarters
EMCA House
23/23-B, Ansari Road, Daryaganj
New Delhi 110 002, India
Landline: +91-11-23272143, +91-11-23272703
+91-11-23282021, +91-11-23245672
E-mail: jaypee@jaypeebrothers.com

Corporate Office
4838/24, Ansari Road, Daryaganj
New Delhi 110 002, India
Phone: +91-11-43574357
Fax: +91-11-43574314
E-mail: jaypee@jaypeebrothers.com

Overseas Office
J.P. Medical Ltd.
83, Victoria Street, London
SW1H 0HW (UK)
Phone: +44-20 3170 8910
E-mail: info@jpmedpub.com

EU GPSR Authorised Representative
Logos Europe, 9 rue Nicolas Poussin
17000, La Rochelle, France
Phone: +33 (0) 6 67 93 73 78
E-mail: contact@logoseurope.eu

Website: www.jaypeebrothers.com
Website: www.jaypeedigital.com

Inquiries for bulk sales may be solicited at: jaypee@jaypeebrothers.com

Emergencies in Otorhinolaryngology

First Edition: 2014
Reprint: **2026**

ISBN: 978-93-5152-105-1

Printed at Replika Press Pvt. Ltd.

Dedicated to

All My Patients Dead or Alive

Contributors

GC Sahoo
Department of ENT
Rajah Muthiah Medical College
Annamalai University
Annamalai Nagar, Tamil Nadu, India

Abhoya Kumar Kar
Formerly HOD of ENT
MKCG Medical College
Berhampur, Odisha, India

Kalpana Dasgupta
HOD of ENT
Akola Medical College
Maharashtra, India

KC Mallick
Associate Professor
Department of ENT
SCB Medical College
Cuttack, Odisha, India

VJ Vikram
Associate Professor
Department of ENT
Institute of Child Health/Madras Medical College, Chennai
Tamil Nadu, India

Santosh Swain
Asst. Professor
Department of ENT
Institute of Medical Sciences and SUM Hospital
Bhubaneswar, Odisha, India

CS Prakash
HOD of Anesthesiology
Rajah Muthiah Medical College
Annamalai University, Annamalai Nagar
Tamil Nadu, India

Foreword

Emergencies in ENT are frequently encountered in the Department of Otorhinolaryngology and Head & Neck Surgery (ORL & HNS), but there is hardly any textbook available exclusively on this important subject for the benefit of medical students and residents in ORL and HNS.

The Medical Council of India has also stressed on starting Trauma and Emergency departments in all the medical colleges of India including post-graduation in Emergency Medicine. Keeping in view all these aspects, this book *Emergencies in Otorhinolaryngology* written by Prof GC Sahoo, Retd Head, Department of ENT and Head and Neck Surgery, Rajah Muthiah Medical College, Annamalai University, Tamil Nadu, India, comprehensively covers all the common emergencies in ENT like Epistaxis, Maxillofacial Trauma, Stridor, Neck Space Infections, Vertigo, Foreign Bodies, Airway Obstruction and Tracheostomy, etc. which are essential for any student of ENT to develop the clinical competency for successful patient management in emergencies. The topics covered are mandatory for problem-based learning and will definitely serve as a guide to the practicing ENT specialists including undergraduate and postgraduate students of ENT.

The author will update in the future edition after getting constructive criticism, valuable opinion, suggestions and feedback from the esteemed readers.

Abhoya Kumar Kar
Formerly HOD of ENT
MKCG Medical College
Berhampur, Odisha, India

Foreword

I congratulate Dr Govind Chandra Sahoo, Ex-Professor and Head of the Department of ENT and Head and Neck Surgery, Rajah Muthiah Medical College, Annamalai University, Annamalai Nagar, Tamil Nadu, India, for writing the book entitled *Emergencies in Otorhinolaryngology*. Prof Sahoo is an eminent academician with 30 years of teaching and clinical experiences. He has reflected all his clinical experiences in this book. Earlier, he has written two books, *MCQs in ENT (2008)* and *History of Medicine (2011)* of international standard.

This book *Emergencies in Otorhinolaryngology* will be highly beneficial for the undergraduate and postgraduate students as well as for ENT specialists working in district headquarters. It will be very rewarding to the author if this book becomes a source of information for all the doctors working in this specialtiy.

Rankanidhi Samal

HOD ENT, IMS and SUM Hospital
Bhubaneswar, Odisha, India

Ex-Professor and HOD ENT
MKCG Medical College
Berhampur, Odisha, India

Preface

Emergency medicine has taken a rapid stride in the last decade or so; but, very few books are written by the authors keeping in mind the needs of both undergraduate and postgraduate medical students which is even more true in the subject of otorhinolaryngology. The author has made an honest attempt to include various aspects of emergencies in the field of ENT along with a few chapters from various contributory authors also, who are experts in their respective fields. A comprehensive chapter on maxillofacial trauma is given, as road traffic accidents causing facial injury and other trauma in head and neck area are increasing every year. It is bound to have some mistakes, omissions, lacunae or drawback in the first edition, but it will be updated after getting the critical remarks from the esteemed readers along with addition of new chapters in subsequent editions.

GC Sahoo

Acknowledgments

I acknowledge with a profound sense of gratitude to the Vice-Chancellor and Registrar of Annamalai University for giving me permission to write and edit this book titled *Emergencies in Otorhinolaryngology*. I also acknowledge the Dean and Medical Superintendent of RMM & H for their constant encouragement to write this manuscript. My special thanks to all the contributory authors for sending their respective chapters well in time; and last but not least, my postgraduate students for whom this book is meant for. I am also grateful to my former postgraduates for excellent typesetting while writing the manuscripts, namely Dr Karthik, Dr Cherrian, Dr Bibin, Dr Senthil Ganesh, Dr Harsha Vardhan, Dr Honey Sebastin, Dr VJ Vikram, Dr Nidhi Mathew, Dr Vinod, Dr John, Dr Abhilash Jayakumar and Dr Vidyadharan, etc. My special thanks to my son Amit Kumar Sahoo and daughter-in-law Snata for doing the cover designing.

Contents

CHAPTER

1 Epistaxis

INTRODUCTION

Epistaxis, or bleeding from the nose, is a common occurrence. The estimated lifetime incidence is 60%, most episodes are minor and do not require intervention or evaluation. Minor bleeding occurs in children and young adults, whereas, severe bleeding, requiring intervention, often occurs in individuals over 50 years of age.

VASCULAR ANATOMY

It is important to understand the blood supply of nose to apply the appropriate treatment. Blood supply to the nasal cavity (both septum and lateral wall) originates from external carotid artery (80%) and internal carotid artery and has multiple anastomoses, most prominent being the Kiesselbach's plexus in the anterior nasal septum.

External Carotid Artery

Its branches are the facial artery and internal maxillary artery (IMA). Superior labial artery is the branch of facial artery which gives branches (septal) near the columella that supply the anterior nasal septum.

The IMA courses through the pterygopalatine fossa and terminates into the sphenopalatine artery (SPA) (artery of epistaxis), which enters the nasal cavity through the sphenopalatine foramen in the lateral nasal wall. The SPA has two main branches on entering the foramen: (1) Nasopalatine artery, supplying the posterior nasal septum and (2) A posterior superior branch, supplying the middle and inferior turbinates. The SPA can divide before entering the foramen. One can have more than 2 branches in the foramen, which should be kept in mind while ligation. The other terminal branch of IMA is the descending palatine artery, which traverses within the greater palatine canal and supplies the anterior septum through the incisive foramen.

Internal Carotid Artery

It divided into anterior ethmoidal and posterior ethmoidal, which are the branches of ophthalmic artery.

These arteries enter the nasal cavity through foramina in the medial orbital wall, within the frontoethomoidal suture. The anterior ethmoidal foramen is located 24 mm posterior to the lacrimal crest. The posterior one is found 12 mm posterior to the anterior one, although the posterior ethmoidal can be absent in 1/3rd of individuals.

The optic nerve is located 6 mm posterior to the posterior ethmoidal artery, if present.

BLOOD SUPPLY

Blood Supply of Nasal Septum (Figure 1.1A)

- Anterior ethmoidal artery
- Sphenopalatine artery
- Septal branches of superior labial artery
- Greater palatine artery

  These 4 arteries form the little's area or Kiesselbach's plexus, at the anteroinferior nasal septum.
- Posterior ethmoidal artery.

Blood Supply of Lateral Wall of Nose (Figure 1.1B)

- Anterior ethmoidal artery
- Posterior ethmoidal artery
- Sphenopalatine artery
- Greater palatine artery.

Woodruff's plexus—venous plexus found in many people in the lateral wall of posteroinferior meatus.

Retrocolumellar vein—runs vertically downwards, just behind the columella, which is a common site of bleeding in the young.

Sites of Epistaxis

- Little's area (90%)
- Woodruff's area
- Septal turbinate
- Nasopharynx
- Diffuse
- Brown's area (posterior part of nasal septum).

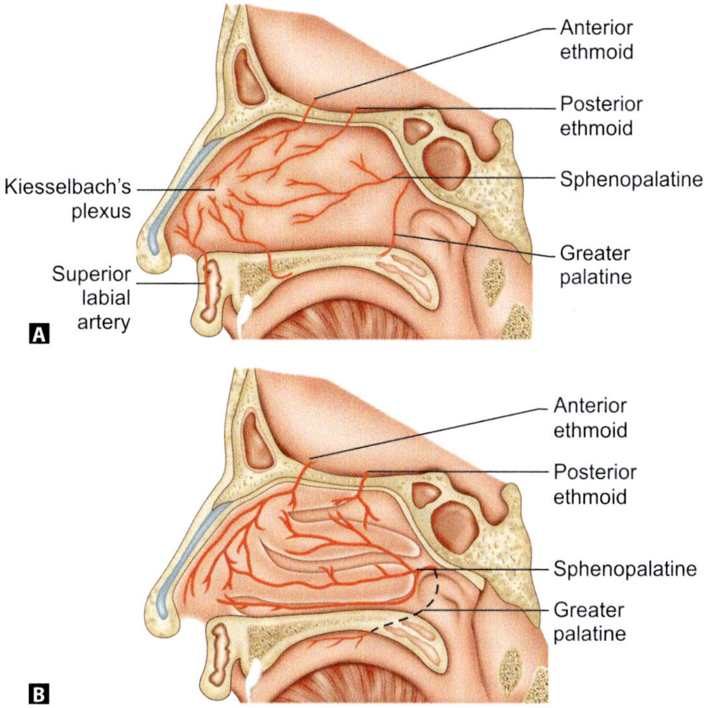

Figures 1.1A and B (A) Blood supply of the nasal septum; (B) Blood supply of the lateral nasal wall

EPIDEMIOLOGY

Epistaxis is extremely common and affects all age groups. Males are slightly more affected than females, although after 50 years of age, the male-female ratio is 1:1. Children and young adults are more often affected with minor episodes of anterior nasal bleeding, whereas the incidence of severe posterior episodes due to hypertension/atherosclerosis is greater in those who are more than 50. It is more common in colder winter months and hot dry climate with low humidity.

Causes of Epistaxis

Local

- Congenital—unilateral choanal atresia
  - Encephalocele
  - Meningocele
  - Glioma
  - Multiple telangiectasis (Osler-Rendu-Weber syndrome)

- Acquired
  - Infective
    - Acute—viral, bacterial, fungal
    - Chronic—specific: TB, syphilis, leprosy; nonspecific—rhinoscleroma
  - Inflammatory
    - Rhinosinusitis (Vasomotor/Allergic)
    - Nasal polyposis
  - Trauma
    - Iatrogenic (Digital trauma)
    - Facial trauma
    - Foreign body
    - Surgery
  - Idiopathic
    - Little's area
    - Woodruff's area
    - Superior part of nose
    - Middle meatus
  - Neoplastic
    - Benign—transitional cell papilloma, angiofibroma (Juvenile Nasopharyngeal Angiofibroma)
    - Malignant—squamous cell carcinoma, adenocarcinoma, adenocystic carcinoma, olfactory neuroblastoma, melanoma, lymphoma
  - Drug induced
    - Rhinitis medicamentosa
  - Inhalants—tobacco, cannabis, heroin, chrome, mercury (Hg), phosphorus, wood dust.

General

- Bleeding disorders
  - Coagulopathies
    - Inherited—coagulation factor deficencies, i.e. factor VIII and IX
    - Acquired—anticoagulants, liver disease, vitamin K deficiency, disseminated intravascular coagulation (DIC), acquired inhibitors of coagulation
  - Platelet disorders
    - Thrombocytopenia—(a) congenital, (b) acquired
    - Marrow failure, i.e. aplasia, drugs, infiltration
    - DIC, hypersplenism, massive blood loss
  - Platelet dysfunction—congenital, Von Willebrand's disease, Bernard-Soulier syndrome, Glanzmann's thrombasthenia

- Acquired
  - Myeloproliferative disease/leukemia/uremia, dysparaproteinemias
  - Drugs—aspirin, NSAIDs
  - Acquired storage pool disease
- Blood vessel disorders
  - Congenital—osteogenesis imperfecta, hereditary hemorrhagic telangiectasia
  - Acquired—amyloid, vasculitis, vitamin C deficiency
- Hyperfibrinolysis
  - Congenital—$\alpha 2$ antiplasmin deficiency
  - Acquired—malignancy, DIC, fibrinolytic therapy
- Drugs
  - Aspirin
  - Anticoagulants
  - Chloramphenicol
  - Methotrexate
  - Immune suppression
  - Alcohol
  - Dipyrimadole
- Neoplasms
- Miscellaneous:
  - Inflammatory disorders
  - Dengue fever
  - Acute exenthematous fevers
  - Wegener's granuloma
  - Extreme heat and cold
  - Vicarious menstruation
  - Sarcoidosis
  - Lethal midline granuloma
- Others
  - Liver failure
  - Hypothyroidism
  - HIV/AIDS
  - Systemic diseases such as hypertension, cirrhosis, chronic nephritis athero-sclerosis, mitral stenosis, etc.

EVALUATION

Once hemodynamic stability and airway patency is confirmed, a quick history taking will identify most of the contributing factors. Laterality of the bleed, amount of blood loss, severity and duration should be ascertained. Presence of nasal obstruction, especially with recurrent bleeding on same side, should be viewed with suspicion. History of nasal trauma should be ruled out. History of medical conditions, medications, alcohol use, severe nose bleeds or easy bruising should be noted. A family history is also asked, for the examination seeks to rule out the predisposing factors and source of bleeding.

Epistaxis is classified operationally into anterior and posterior. Anterior epistaxis is the bleeding arising from the more anterior vessels and posterior epistaxis from the posterior vessels. Such a classification helps to define which treatment option will likely be necessary. Examination starts with anterior rhinoscopy. Significant hemorrhage will require suction, a light source, nasal speculum and an endoscope, care is taken while manipulating the clots, since they can cause aspiration.

Supplies and Equipment for the Evaluation and Treatment of Epistaxis in the Urgent Care Setting

- Personal protective supplies
  - Mask
  - Gown
  - Eye protection
- Wall suction and tubing
- Frazier tip suctions, size 10 and 12 French
- Headlight
- Nasal speculum
- Bayonet forceps
- Cotton or neurosurgical cottonoid sponges
- Silver nitrate cautery sticks
- Packing materials
  - Merocel nasal sponges (Merocel Corporation)
  - Vaseline strip gauze (Sherwood Medical)
  - Gelfoam (Upjohn Company)
  - Surgical (Johnson and Johnson)
- Suction cautery unit
- 0 and 30 degree rigid nasal endoscopes with light source
- Optical loupe magnification
- Vasoconstrictors and anesthetics
  - 4% xylocaine
  - 0.5% to 1% phenylephrine
  - 2% topical lidocaine solution
  - 1% injectable lidocaine with 1:100,000 epinephrine
- Antibiotic ointment (without neomycin)
- Tongue blades, two 10-cc syringes with IS- and 27-gauge needles.

Laboratory Studies

These should be done in recurrent or severe cases. A complete blood count, APPT platelet count, bleeding time, prothrombin time, partial thromboplastin time should be done. Hepatic and renal indices should also be investigated.

Imaging Studies

These include CT scan (with or without contrast), MRI, angiography, and chest X-ray. Diagnostic angiography, if embolization is chosen as the treatment modality.

Treatment

- Hemodynamic stability and intravenous access with airway patency should be assured
- Blood transfusion, if necessary, may also be warranted.

Medical Management

Aim

- To stem anterior/posterior bleed
- To improve visualization during examination.

Drugs

- Topical vasoconstrictors like 1% phenylephrine or 0.05% oxymetazoline are commonly used
- Topical anesthetic agents like 2–4% lidocaine.

Anterior Epistaxis

Cauterization

- Chemical cauterization—silver nitrate stickers can be applied to the anesthetized nasal septum with minimal discomfort. Cauterization should be limited to one side of the septum, or separated by 4 to 6 weeks to avoid perforation. It is useful in minor bleeds
- Electrocauterization—useful for more aggressive bleeds. The anesthetized site is cauterized conservatively to avoid perforation. More posterior bleeds require endoscopy
- Laser cauterization—more useful in chronic patients with hereditary hemorrhagic telangiectasia. Potassium titanyl phosphate or CO_2 lasers are used. They have little role.

Nasal Packing (Anterior)

This is the next option if medical management and cautery fails. Absorbable and non-absorbable materials are available for packing (Figures 1.2A and B).

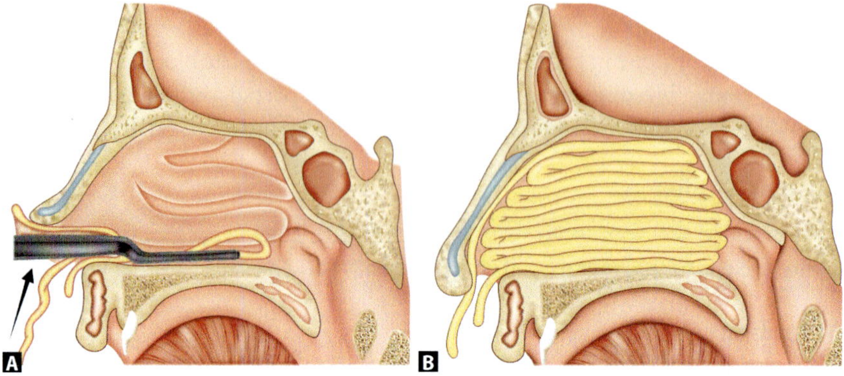

Figures 1.2A and B Placement of traditional anterior nasal packing

Absorbable Packs

- Oxidized cellulose
- Gelatin foam

  These two encourage platelet aggregation, tamponade the site, protect the mucosa from drying and trauma.
- Floseal—it is a thrombin-gelatin product
- BIPP (Bismuth iodine paraffin pack).

Advantages

- Ease of application
- Comfortable
- Confirms to the irregular contours of nasal cavity
- Less painful
- More effective in the emergency room patients, for initial control of epistaxis.

Nonabsorbable Packs

- Inflatable balloons
- Carboxymethyl cellulose sponges
- Calcium alginate
- Petroleum jelly impregnated gauze.

Disadvantages

- Patient discomfort
- Need for removal (can be kept for 1–5 days)
- Patient needs to be put on antibiotics to prevent toxic-shock syndrome. The pack can be coated with antibiotic ointment.

Complications

Ulcerations, septal perforation, sinusitis, synechiae, hypoxemia, arrhythmias.

Ligation of Ethmoidal Vessels

Anterior ethmoidal artery cannot be embolized due to risk of blindness or stroke. Surgical ligation is done by:

- Lynch incision: Periosteum is raised off the lacrimal crest and posteriorly into the orbit. The artery is clipped or coagulated by bipolar electrocauterization
- Transnasal endoscopic approach through lamina papyracea, has recently been described.

Posterior Epistaxis

This most likely originates from the SPA and posterior ethmoidal artery (PEA), although rare.

The main methods of treatment include:

1. Endoscopic cauterization (electro)
2. Posterior nasal packing
3. Embolization
4. Surgical arterial ligation.

Endoscopic Cauterization

Endoscopic cauterization was successfully employed in 81% of the cases. The most common site was the lateral nasal wall. Posterior nasal cauterization often requires general anesthesia and a thorough examination with rigid endoscopes.

Posterior Nasal Packing

It is not used as frequently as anterior and is more risky. The various packs are:

- Those with anterior and posterior balloons, with separate ports for differential inflation pressures
- Foley's catheter (12 to 14 FG) (Figure 1.3)—after placing it into the nasal cavity, the balloon is inflated with 5–10 mL saline and placed anteriorly so that the balloon is lodged at the choanas. An anterior pack is kept in conjunction. It should be secured at the nasal sill to maintain pressure. Padding should be used to protect the alar and columella, to prevent pressure necrosis.

Complications

Ulcerations, septal perforation, sinusitis, synechiae, hypoxemia, arrythmias, alar, columellar or palatal necrosis, apnea, hypoxia, dysrhythmia. Patients with posterior packs should be admitted for inpatient care with pulse oximetry and oxygen supplied, as needed.

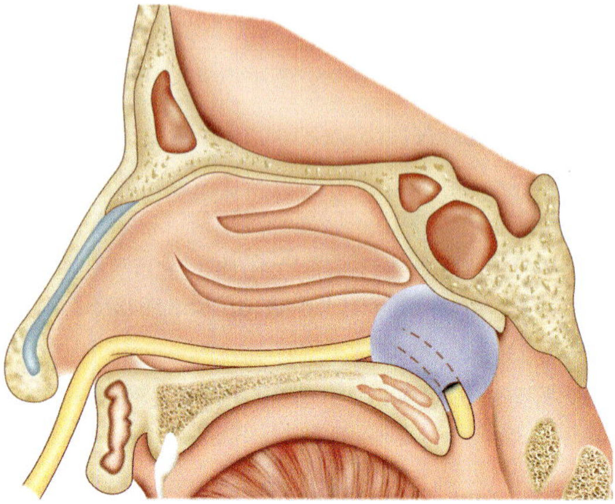

Figure 1.3 Positioning of a balloon (Foley's catheter) posterior pack

Embolization

The common embolization targets are IMA and facial artery.

The various materials used for embolization are cyanoacrylate glue, polyvinyl alcohol sponge, metal coils, and gelatin foam. Success rate range from 79–96%.

Complications

- Rebleeding
- Stroke
- Blindness
- Facial numbness
- Skin sloughing
- Carotid artery dissection
- Groin hematoma.

Drawbacks

- Expensive
- Inability to control bleed from ethmoidal arteries.

Surgical Ligation

- IMA ligation

  The approach is similar to a Caldwell-LUC's operation, with access into the pterygomaxillary fossa, through the posterior maxillary wall. The IMA is then identified and clipped or electrocauterized.

  Complications—sinusitis, facial and gum numbness and oroantral fistula

- External carotid artery ligation

  It may be considered for cases of refractory bleeding. Procedure is performed under local or general anesthesia. At least, two branches of the artery should be identified before ligation. Complications include injury to hypoglossal, vagal and superior laryngeal nerves.
- Transnasal Endoscopic SPA Ligation (TESPAL)
  - Performed under local or general anesthesia
  - Nose is adequately decongested topically and the SPA is injected with lidocaine and epinephrine through the greater palatine foramen
  - A 0° 4 mm nasal endoscope is used to see the posterior portion of the middle turbinate and its attachment
  - A 10–20 mm incision is made vertically, 5 mm anterior to the middle turbinate attachment
  - A mucosal flap is raised posteriorly until the crista ethmoidalis is reached
  - The SPA is identified posterior to this landmark
  - It is then clipped or electrocauterized
  - Results range from 87–100%.

Complications

Palatal numbness, sinusitis, decreased lacrimation, septal perforation, and necrosis of inferior turbinate. Given its high success rate, this procedure has become the treatment of choice in posterior epistaxis.

Septoplasty

Patients with epistaxis, thought to be a result of a deviated septum leading to drying and excoriation of the mucosa may benefit from septoplasty.

SUMMARY

Epistaxis is a common problem that ranges from a minor nuisance to a life-threatening emergency. Multiple modalities exist for treatment and sometimes more than one should be used. Surgeons should be prepared to deal with severe or refractory bleeding through the use of the medication, packing and radiological or surgical methods. Identifying the likely source of the bleeding, based on a thorough knowledge of the vascular anatomy, increases the likelihood of a successful treatment.

BIBLIOGRAPHY

1. Weiss NS. Relation of high blood pressure to headache, epistaxis, and selected other symptoms. The United States Health Examination Survey of Adults. N Engl J Med. 1972; 287:361-3.

2. Massick D, Tobin EJ. Epistaxis. In: Cummings CW, Haughey BH, Thomas JR, et al. (Ed) Cummings Otolarynagology: Head and Neck Surgery. Philadelphia: Mosby: 2005. P. 942- 61.
3. Floreani SR, Nair SB, Switajewski MC, et al. Endoscopic anterior ethmodidal artery ligation: a cadaver study. Laryngoscope. 2006;116:1263-7.
4. Tan LK, Calhoun KH, Epistaxis. Med Vlin North Am. 1999;83:43-56.
5. Wormadl PJ. Epistaxis. In: Bailey BJ, Calhoun KH, Derkay C, et al. (Ed) Head and Neck Surgry–Otolaryngology. Philadephila: Lippincott Williams & Wilkins; 2006. P. 505-14.
6. Orlandi RR, Lanza DC. Is nasal packing necessary following endoscopic sinus surgery? Laryngoscope. 2004;114(9):1541-4.
7. Douglas R. Wormald PJ. Pterygopalatine fossa infiltration through the greater palatine foramen: where to bend the needle. Laryngoscope. 2006;116(7):1255-7.
8. Hanif J, Tasca RA, Frosh A, et al. Silver nitrate: histological effects of cautery on epithelial surfaces with vrying contact times. Clin Otolaryngol Allied Sco. 2003;28(4):368-70.
9. Aassar OS, Friedman CM, White RI. The natural history of epistaxis in hereditary hemorrhagic elangiectasia, Laryngoscope. 1991;101:977.
10. Cannon CR. Effective treatment protocol for posterior epistaxis: a 10-year experience. Otolaryngol Head Neck Surg. 1993;109:722-5.
11. Cullen MM, Tami TA. Comparison of internal maxillary artery ligation versus embolizaiton for refractory posterior epistaxis. Otolaryngol Head Neck Surg. 1995;113:674.
12. Emanual, JM. Epistaxis. In: cuming CW and others, (Ed). Otolaryngology–Head & Neck Surgry, 3rd Edn., St Louis, Mosby, 1998; pp. 858-78.
13. Harries PG, et al. Treatment of hereditary hemorrhagic telangectasia by the pulsed dye laser. J Laryngol Otol. 1997;111:1038.
14. Jacobs JR, et al. Posterior packs and the nasopulmonary reflex. Laryngoscope. 1981;91:279.
15. Jacobs JR, etal. New Approaches to the Management of Epistaxis: Maintenance Manual for Lifelong Learning, Kendall–Hunt, 2002.

CHAPTER

2 Stridor in Children

Stridor is characterized by harsh, high-pitched musical sound produced by turbulent airflow through the upper airway. Evaluation must be tailored to the clinical situation, and stridor can range from mild to severe to life-threatening. In the later scenario, urgent decision making and treatment are required.

PHYSIOLOGY

Larynx is a complex evolutionary structure that permits the trachea and the bronchi to be joined to the pharynx as a common aerodigestive pathway. The larynx serves the essential functions of:

- Ventilation of the lungs
- Protection of the lungs during deglutition by its sphincter mechanisms
- Clearance of secretions by a vigorous cough
- Vocalization.

An infant's survival is predicated on the structural and neurologic integrity of the larynx and prompt diagnostic and surgical interventions for airway management is mandatory (Figure 2.1).

PATHOPHYSIOLOGY

As relates to any system of tubular fluid dynamics, flow within the system is related to the radius of the tube to the fourth power according to Poiseuille law [$\phi = \pi d^4$] $(P_1 - P_2)/128\ \eta\ L$ (ϕ = volumetric flow note; d = diameter, P = pressure; η = viscocity; L = length of the tube. This law explains why even a minor obstruction in the airway is potentially more significant for a child than for an adult. The other physical law that is crucial to a proper understanding of a pediatric stridor is the Bernouilli law, which states that as velocity increases through a constant area, the pressure on the wall of the lumen decreases (W = PAV; W = work, P = pressure, A = area, V = velocity).

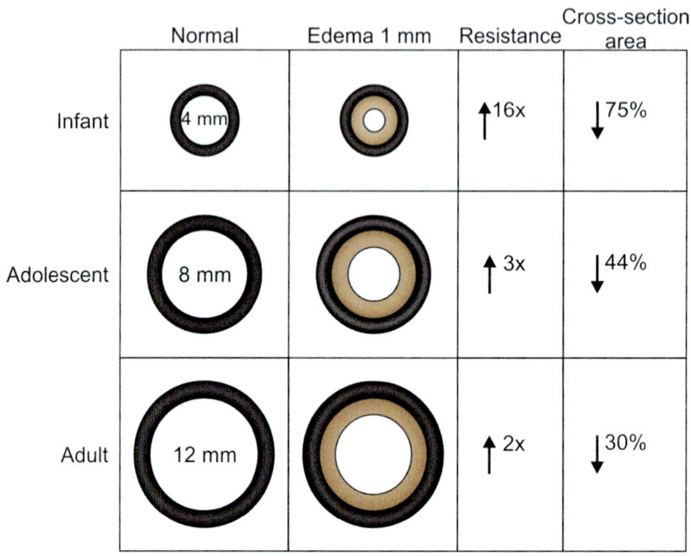

Figure 2.1 Laryngeal inlet cross-sectional area in normal and laryngeal edema

In other words, airflow dynamics dispose a region, where these is an anatomic narrowing to collapse further, dynamically, with increased turbulent airflow through that region. The resulting stridor can be localized to discrete areas of the airway according to the nature of the sound in relationship to the phase of breathing.

These discrete regions can be divided into three zones (Table 2.1):

- A supraglottic and supralaryngeal zone (including the pharynx)
- An extrathoracic tracheal zone (including both glottis and subglottis)
- An intrathoracic tracheal zone (including primary and secondary bronchus).

Supraglottic lesions often cause stridor during inspiration, whereas lesions of the intrathoraic trachea (or) bronchi are aggravated during expiration.

Table 2.1 Obstructive symptoms and their relationship to site of obstruction

Location	*Voice*	*Stridor*	*Retraction*	*Feeding*	*Cough*
Laryngeal supraglottic	Muffled Hot potato	Snoring Inspiratory Fluttering	None until late obstruction	Difficult to impossible	Not noted
Laryngeal subglottic	Normal occasionally hoarse	Inspiratory-expiratory snoring	Intercostal early, then xyphoid	Normal	Barking
Tracheal	Normal	Expiratory and wheezing	None, except in severe obstruction	Normal	Brassy

The first zone, which is composed of the supraglottis, tongue and pharynx, is relatively loosely supported and often falls into the airway (or) it drawn into it during inspiration. Inspiration is initiated by the expansion of the thorax, lung tissue and intrathoracic branches. Stridor, for this zone, is generally inspiratory and high-pitched.

The second (or) extrathoracic trachea is a neutral zone affected equally by both inspiration and expiration. The vocal ligament tightly supports the vocal cords between the thyroid and arytenoids cartilages and in the absence of neural stimulation, is rigid. Similarly, the subglottic region is unyielding because of the cricoid ring. Airflow is regulated by absolute lumen size, because the airway cannot contract (or) expand dynamically.

When stridor develops in this zone, the glottis and subglottis lumen has reached critically smaller diameter. Stridor produced in this region is often biphasic, being heard during both inspiration and expiration and is of intermediate pitch.

In the third (or) intrathroracic bronchial zone, exhalation commences by the contraction of the thorax. As air moves during expiration, the Bernoulli's principle again adds a constricting force. The resultant sound is expiratory in nature and less harsh than stridor but retains a musical quality and is often called wheeze.

INITIAL HISTORY AND EVALUATION

Evaluation of a child with stridor requires a carefully taken history and thorough physical examination, as well as, knowledge of the functional anatomy of the upper airway. Stridor may result from obstruction of one of the several sites in the upper airway.

CASES OF STRIDOR IN CHILDREN ACCORDING TO SITE OF OBSTRUCTION

Pharynx

- Congenital anomalies
  - Lingual thyroid
  - Choanal atresia
  - Craniofacial anomalies (Apert syndrome, Robin syndrome)
  - Cysts (dermoid).

Inflammatory

- Abscess (parapharyngeal, retropharyngeal)
- Diphtheria.

Larynx

- Congenital anomalies
    - Laryngomalacia
    - Webs, cysts, laryngocele
    - Cartilage dystrophy
    - Subglottic stenosis
    - Cri-du-chat syndrome.

Inflammatory

- Epiglottis
- Croup.

Miscellaneus

- Foreign body
- Laryngismus stridulus.

Vocal Cord Paralysis

Trauma

- Intubation
- Neck trauma
- Burn and scald injury.

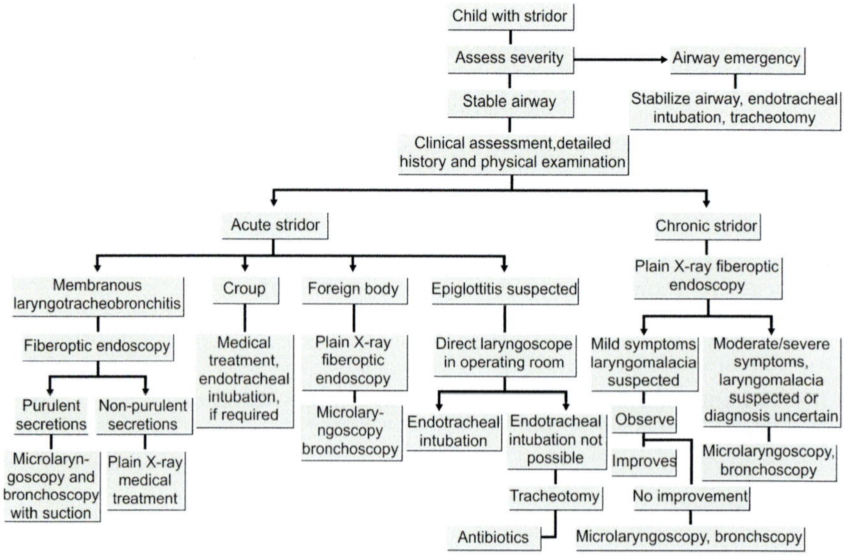

Figure 2.2 Algorithm of stridor managment

Neoplasm

- Subglottic hemangioma
- Laryngeal papilloma
- Cystic hygroma
- Laryngeal cancer.

ASSESSMENT

History

The obstetric and perinatal histories are often relevant, especially if the child was born prematurely and required ventilation. Few neonates older than 32 weeks of gestation will require ventilation for respiratory distress syndrome, with ventilation becoming a virtual certainly in neonates younger than 28 weeks, even with the administration of surfactant.

Stridor that is present at birth with the child's first breath, is unusual and generally denotes a fixed congenital narrowing such as laryngeal web, subglottic stenosis (or) tracheal narrowing. Dynamic conditions such as laryngomalacia becomes evident in the first few weeks of life. The stridor in congenital vocal cord palsy is increasing as it often presents immediately postpartum, suggesting that it may be more an incoordination than a true paralysis.

Stridor is seldom constant and any diural or other variation can help pinpoint the cause, although asking parents about the timing of any stridor in the cycle, is seldom profitable. Typically, laryngomalacia is better with the child at rest and asleep but made worse by crying, feeding and when distressed.

Airway obstruction produces a number of associated symptoms alongside stridor including recession, apnea, cyanosis, "dying spells" dyspnea, tachypnea, cough and hoarseness. Apneas with cyanosis are typical of severe tracheomalacia and are sometimes termed dying spells. Tachypnea and dyspnea are not limited to upper airway obstruction, but a clear description of exertional dyspnea in an older child provides a useful functional assessment of severity. Cough is typical of tracheoesophageal fistula and tracheomalacia and is rarely because of "infant asthma".

Feeding is closely connected with breathing, particularly in the infant and an accurate picture of the feeding pattern must be obtained. Breastfed babies with airway obstruction will characteristically "come up for air" whereas bottle-fed babies may require thickened feeds or a "slow teat" (i.e. one with small holes).

EXAMINATION

A general impression can be obtained while taking the history but a careful general examination is necessary to avoid nursing subtle features of related syndromes (or) of other general pediatric disease.

Observing the child at rest provides not only an initial assessment of the degree of respiratory distress but also the characteristics of any stridor. Typically, inspiratory stridor is because of an intrathoracic obstruction from the larynx or high trachea with branchial or low tracheal obstruction producing an expiratory stridor. Biphasic stridor can occur with obstruction anywhere in the tracheobronchial tree. Even if expiratory stridor is absent, a prolonged phase may be present indicating an intrathoracic obstruction. The characteristic sound of stridor, even in a common condition such as laryngomalacia is so variable as to be of little diagnostic use of its own.

Subcostal, intercostal suprasternal recession may occur separately or together and can also be associated with see-saw respiration. Cyanosis is a late event and no comfort should be taken from the fact that a child still looks pink.

Both stridor and recession will vary as the child rests, cries and sleeps, but it is rare to be able to demonstrate on similar repeatable with position. Observing the child feeding is very valuable, particularly if poor feeding (or) aspiration is a significant feature in the history.

PRE-ENDOSCOPY INVESTIGATIONS

In acute airway obstruction, O_2 saturation monitoring is extremely helpful as it is noninvasive (unlike arterial blood gases) and yet much more sensitive than clinical estimation as cyanosis is a very late event. Desaturation occurs with tiredness, more often than progression of the underlying obstruction. CO_2 builds up and develop without destruction, especially if O_2 is being administered.

Tosterin and others have reviewed the value of radiological investigation retrospectively. A plain chest X-ray and a Cincinnati view are appropriate screening investigations with further radiographs, such as contrast studies. A plain chest X-ray may show the ground glass appearance of bronchopulmonary dysplasia (or) mediastinal shift with obstructive emphysema of a foreign body. If a foreign body is suspected, a more sensitive technique is diaphragmatic screening with video fluoroscopy in young children and inspiratory and expiratory films in older children to demonstrate diaphragmatic immobility on the side of the obstruction.

Bronchography is enjoying something of a renaissance after the introduction of safer nonionic contrast media. It is particularly useful for the lower airway, demonstrating tracheobrachial stenosis and malacia. Opening pressures of the collapsed bronchi and lower trachea can be measured and used to determine the level of airway support needed.

Pediatric lung function tests are seldom used, because more children in whom there is doubt about the relative contribution of upper and lower airway components are too young to perform the tests.

Computed tomography (CT) and the magnetic resonance imaging (MRI) are not usually sufficiently-sensitive to fully characterize a stenotic segment, which can be more accurately assessed at endoscopy. If available, helical CT with multiplanar reconstruction may offer better definition of tracheal lesion. MRI and CT scan, however, both demonstrate extrinsic compression, particularly abnormal vasculature.

Gastroesophageal reflux can be assessed with a contrast study, pH probe study or lower esophageal biopsy. Contrast Studies have low specificity and sensitivity and are very dependent on the radiologist for appropriate positioning and interpretation. The laryngologist is interested in the pH in the upper esophagus and pharynx, which can be measured using a second probe in the upper esophagus. Double probe pH studies are at present more than that of a research tool because of technical difficulties with the probe and little in the way of normative date.

Ultrasound of vocal cords can be used to demonstrate vocal cord palsy with reasonable accuracy to complement the endoscopic findings. Transcutaneous electromyography (EMG) is helpful in the adults, especially if the nerve has been severed.

A sleep study is rarely used in the assessment of the stridulous child, as airway obstruction that worsens during sleep, is usually a feature of pharyngeal obstruction.

Lung function tests such as flow volume loops will help localize the site of obstruction but do require a degree of patient cooperation.

FLEXIBLE ENDOSCOPY IN THE OFFICE OR WARD

The introduction of ultrathin endoscopes with good optics and a diameter of less than 2 mm have allowed even neonates to be endoscoped without the need for a general anesthetic.

Performing an endoscopy in the ward, using a flexible scope and no anesthesia, is particularly useful in assessing dynamic abnormalities such as vocal cord palsy, before a formal endoscopy in the operating room.

LARYNGOTRACHEOBRONCHOSCOPY

Laryngotracheobronchoscopy is the gold standard in the assessment of the stridulous child. The advent of video has been invaluable in training and has made assessment safer, because the anesthetist can now monitor the endoscopy as the screen and the nurse can be ready with equipment for the next stage.

The latest digital image recording systems allow multiple rapid images to be stored during the procedure with only a selected few being printed either on polaroid or converted to slide format. As computer memory becomes even more affordable, digital video recordings, as well as still images can be saved and archived.

Anesthetic

As atropine, premedication offers a dry surgical field and also improves the efficacy of typical anesthetic, but to be effective it needs to be given by intramuscular injection. Intravenous induction is preferable for older children, although gas induction may be needed in the infants. Intravenous succinylcholine can be given, if the patient is stable to avoid laryngeal spasm.

Intubation

Once intubated, the child can be quickly ventilated down to a level of anesthesia that will allow the passage of endoscopes without gagging but maintains spontaneous respiration.

Jet Ventilation

This technique allows the child to be paralyzed, preventing any coughing or gagging. Gas exchange is maintained, however, with short pulses of injected anesthetic gas, simulating normal respiration.

Laryngeal Mask

This is useful for fiberoptic bronchoscopy, particularly, if the patient is difficult to intubate because of mandibular hypoplasia.

Microlaryngoscopy

A small sandbag is usually required under the shoulder to prevent hyperextension of the neck.

A 30° telescope should be in hand to assess the supraglottic larynx without splinting. A microscope should be available. If a microscope is used, a 400 mm lens allows the use of standard laryngeal instruments, but a 350 mm lens brings the patient closer, allowing easier manipulation of larynx.

Laryngeal examination usually begins with the endotracheal tube in place by gently inserting the lubricated suspension laryngoscope, taking care to protect the teeth and lips and to keep the tongue central to provide a well-centered view. As in adults, it is important to check the overall appearance of the supraglottis and laryngopharynx during introduction of the laryngoscope.

Laryngeal examination with the endotracheal tube removed, provides a superior view, by using a probe to move the arytenoids independently. The mobility of the cricoarytenoid joints can be assessed. If an interarytenoid scar is present, the arytenoids will not move independently. A posterior laryngeal cleft is excluded by passing the probe between the arytenoids, comparing the lower limit of the interarytenoid groove with that of the posterior commissure. Finally, the cords need to be gently moved apart to affect the subglottis.

Bronchoscopy

An appropriate-sized bronchoscope is used. Unless stenosis is suspected neonate pose particular problems if manipulation of the airway is required. An anesthetic laryngoscope can be used in the vallecula to lift the larynx forward while passing the level of the bronchoscope through the vocal cords under video control on the monitor. The main bronchi, the carina, the trachea and the subglottis are all systematically examined and videographs (or) digital images recorded.

DYNAMIC ASSESSMENT OF LARYNX ON RECOVERY FROM ANESTHESIA

Dynamic assessment of the vocal cord movement is to insert a laryngeal mask, a fiberoptic bronchoscope passed through this to just above the laryngeal inlet. If a bilateral vocal cord palsy is suspected and structural abnormalities have been excluded with a full microlaryngoscopy and rigid bronchoscope. An alternative is to use a 30-degree scope, which gives a view of the larynx without splitting the supraglottis.

TREATMENT OF ACUTE AIRWAY OBSTRUCTION

Medical

For example, a child arriving in the emergency room with suspected laryngotracheobronchitis (LTB). There is no objective evidence that raising the humidity of the inspired air is beneficial, however, many units still use humidity tents (or) "Croupette" that have the disadvantage of decreased visibility as well as doing little, to allay the fear of frightened child.

Intravenous (and oral) steroids such as dexamethasone have been shown to be beneficial in croups (LTB) with inhaled steroids having a similar effect.

All children with croup symptoms who demonstrate increased wake of breathing in the clinics (or) emergency departments should be treated with glucocorticoids. This treatment may be nebulized budesonide (2 mg) or IM dexamethasone (dose may be 0.15–0.6 mg/kg). Oral dexamethasone may be the best option because of its ease of administration, wide spread availability and lower cost. L-epinephrine (5 mL of 1:1000) or racemic epinephrine (0.5 mL) should be considered for children with croup who have moderate (or) severe distress.

Management of the Difficult to Extubate Neonate

- Treat reflux
- Leave tube in place for at least 1 week between trials of extubation
- Steroids to cover extubation
- Nasal prongs with CPAP postextubation
- Endoscopy with laser for small granulation, cysts and so on
- Cricoid split
- Single-stage laryngeal reconstruction
- Tracheostomy with stent to maintain airway.

Cricoid Split

This operation is designed to decompress the complete cricoid ring and expand the lumen without grafting.

Cricoid split in indicated in neonates who fail extubation because of subglottic edema or soft immature stenosis. It is contraindicated in patients who weigh less than 1.5 kg and those with other medical problems, particularly an oxygen requirement of greater than 35% because of bronchopulmonary dysplasia. The operation consists of a midline laryngofissure from the first tracheal ring to half way up the thyroid cartilage.

Postoperative intubation lasts usually for a week and this rest period is probably important in the success of the operation. Long-term paralysis produces lung atelectasis of neuromuscular weakness, which should be avoided.

Single Stage Laryngeal Reconstruction

In premature neonates, who fail extubation, single-stage laryngeal reconstruction is indicated as an alternative to tracheostomy, if a mature subglottic stenosis is present.

The operation consists of a midline laryngofissure with an incision from first tracheal ring to halfway up the thyroid cartilage, which then allows reintubation with an age-appropriate tube (or) a tube one size larger. Cartilage is harvested from the rib or ear and carved into a boat shape with beveled edges for security. Postoperatively, the patient is intubated and maintained with minimal sedation and no paralysis for 5 to 10 days (longer if patient is young).

Recent Techniques to Avoid Tracheotomy

- Subglottic stenosis
  - Active medical management
  - Balloon dilation
  - Cricoid split
  - Single-stage laryngotracheoplasty
- Subglottic hemangioma
  - Systemic or intralesional steroids
  - Surgical excision
- Laryngomalacia
  - Aryepiglottoplasty
- Tracheobronchomalacia
  - Continuous positive airway
  - Pressure via endotracheal or tracheotomy tube
  - Intraluminal stents.

BIBLIOGRAPHY

1. Abramson AL, et al. Clinical effects of photodynamic therapy on recurrent laryngeal papillomas. Arch Otolaryngol Head Neck Surg. 1992;118:25.
2. Arnold JE. Advances in pediatric flexible brochoscopy. Otolaryngol Clin. North Am. 1989;22:545.
3. Baraka A, Choneiry P, Medawwar A. The layyngeal mask airway for fiberoptic bronchoscopy in children. Paediatr Anaesth. 1995;5:197.
4. Benjamin B, Carter P. Congenital laryngeal hemangioma. Ann Otol Rhino Laryngol. 1983;92:157.
5. Brodsky L, Yoshpe N, Ruben RJ. Clinicopathological correlates of congenital subglottic hemangiomas. Ann Otol Rhinol Laryngol. 1983;92:4.
6. Burton DM, et al. Pediatric airway manifestation of gastroesophagel reflux. Ann Otol Rhino laryngel. 1992;10:742.
7. Catalona PJ, et al. New approaches to the management of airway obstruction in "high risk" neonates. Arch Otolargngol Head Neck Surg. 1992;118:306.
8. Choa DI, et al. Subglottic hemangioma in children. J laryngol Otol. 1986;100:443.
9. Cohen SR, et al. Laryngeal paralysis in children: a long-term retrospective study. Ann Otol Rhino Laryngol. 1982;91:407.
10. Cole RR, Myer CM III, Cotton KT. Tracheotomy in children with recurrent respiratory papillomatosis, Head Neck. 1989;11:226.
11. Contencin P, et al. Gastroesophageal reflux and ENT disorder in childhood, Int J Pediatr Otorhinlaryrngol. (Suppl.) 1995;35:S135.
12. Cotton RT, Evan JN. Laryrgotracheal reconstruction in children. Five–year follow up. Ann Otol Rhinolaryngol. 1981;90:516.
13. Couser RJ, et al. Effectiveness of dexamethasone in preventing extubation failure in preterm infants at increased risk for airway edema. J Pediatr. 1992;12:591-6.
14. Dawson KP, Steinberg A, Capaldi N. The latest radiograph of neck in laryngotrachea–bronchitis (Croup). J Qual Clin Pract. 1994;14:39.
15. de Blic J, Delacourt C, Scheinmann P. Ultra thin flexible bronchoscopy in neonatal intensive care units. Arch Dis Child. 1991;66(12):1383-5.
16. de Gaudemar L, et al. Outcome of laryngeal paralysis in neonates: a long term retrospective study of 113 cases. Int J Pediator Otorhinolaryngol. 1996;34:101.

CHAPTER

3 Deep Neck Space Infections

Deep neck infections (DNIs) or deep neck space infections are unique among infectious diseases for their versatility and potential for severe complications. Complex head and neck anatomy often makes early recognition of DNIs challenging and a high index of suspicion is necessary to avoid any delay in treatment. Low socioeconomic status and poor oral hygiene have been associated with higher rates of odontogenic infections, including Ludwig's angina.

ANATOMY

Multiple layers of cervical fascia encase the contents of the neck and form the potential head and neck spaces. These fascial planes constitute important anatomical limitations for the spread of infection. The superficial cervical fascia underlies the skin of the head and neck in a continuous plane and covers adipose tissue, sensory nerves, superficial vessels (including the external jugular vein), lymphatics, the platysma muscle and the muscles of facial expression. It extends from the superior aspect of the head down to the shoulders, axilla and thorax and includes the superficial musculoaponeurotic system. It may serve as an additional barrier for containing edema and pressure caused by infections in the underlying muscular and visceral compartments of the neck. Infections can lead to cellulitis and further to abscess formation. A superficial abscess can be drained with a transverse incision along Langer's lines over the area of prominence and cellulitis and abscess should be managed with appropriate antibiotic therapy.

The deep cervical fascia is divided into three layers (superficial, middle and deep) that envelop the contents of the head and neck and form the potential deep neck spaces.

The superficial layer of deep cervical fascia surrounds the neck as it courses from the posterior spinous processes of the vertebrae to its anterior insertions into the sternum, hyoid, mandible and zygomatic arches. It splits to envelop the trapezius and sternocleidomastoid, anterior belly of the digastrics and masseter, submandibular and parotid, and parotid and masticator spaces. Just deep to the sternocleidomastoid (SCM), it contributes to the lateral aspect of the carotid sheath. The anterior- superior aspect of the superficial layer of deep cervical fascia forms the floor of the submandibular spaces as it covers the anterior belly of the digastrics and mylohyoid muscles.

The middle layer of deep cervical fascia encloses the anterior contents of the neck and has two divisions. The muscular division surrounds the sternothyroid, sternohyoid and thyrohyoid and extends from the hyoid bone down to the sternum, clavicle and scapulae. The visceral division envelops the trachea, larynx, pharynx, esophagus and the thyroid gland that lies posterior to the strap muscles and extends from the pharyngeal constrictor muscles and hyoid bone down to the anterior mediastinum overlying the fibrous pericardium and great vessels. The posterior-superior aspect of the middle layer of deep cervical fascia, also known as the buccopharyngeal fascia, courses around the posterior pharynx and forms the anterior wall of the retropharyngeal space.

The deep layer of deep cervical fascia encloses the posterior contents of the neck. It originates along the vertebral spinous processes and courses anteriorly beneath the trapezius muscle while surrounding the deep neck musculature and vertebral column. It divides as it reaches the longus colli muscle and anterior aspect of the vertebral bodies to form the prevertebral fascia and the alar fascia. The alar fascia also serves as the anterior boundary of the danger space, which extends downward into the posterior mediastinum to the level of the diaphragm. Posteriorly, the prevertebral fascia adheres directly to the vertebral bodies and cervical muscles and serves as posterior wall of the danger space. The prevertebral space lies between the vertebral bodies and prevertebral fascia and extends from the skull base down to the coccyx. The prevertebral fascia also envelops the brachial plexus, phrenic nerve, vertebral vessels and subclavian vessels inferiorly and eventually gives rise to the axillary sheath.

The carotid sheath receives connective tissue contributions from all three layers of deep cervical fascia and yet it remains anatomically independent as a barrier against the spread of infection into the carotid space from the adjacent deep neck compartments, of which the parapharyngeal space is the most intimately associated. The carotid sheath protects all the carotid arteries, internal jugular veins, cervical sympathetic chains and cranial nerves IX, X, XI and XII.

DEEP NECK SPACES

At least 11 deep neck spaces lie within the complex framework formed by the cervical fascial planes and they functionally contain DNIs as long as their natural points of resistance along communicating fascial boundaries are not overcome. Anteriorly, strong fascial attachments to the hyoid bone are an important barrier to downward infectious spread. As a result, the deep neck spaces are often classified into three anatomic groups, based on their relation to the hyoid bone:

- Those located above the level of the hyoid bone (peritonsillar, submandibular, parapharyngeal, masticator/temporal, buccal and parotid spaces)
- Those involving the entire length of the neck (retropharyngeal, danger, prevertebral and carotid spaces)
- The anterior visceral or pretracheal space located below the hyoid bone.

Spaces Above the Level of the Hyoid Bone

Peritonsillar Space

The peritonsillar space lies between the palatine tonsil and the adjacent superior pharyngeal constrictor muscle and is bounded anteriorly and posteriorly by the tonsillar pillars. It contains loose continuous tissue. The peritonsillar space is anatomically contiguous with several deeper spaces and peritonsillar infections can potentially involve the parapharyngeal and retropharyngeal spaces. The presence of severe trismus suggests parapharyngeal space and medial pterygoid muscle involvement. Infections limited to the peritonsillar space often present with fever, sore throat, dysphagia, odynophagia, a muffled "hot potato" voice and cervical adenopathy. Examination of the oropharynx may reveal tonsillar edema, visible exudates, bulging of the superior pole of the tonsillar pillar and deviation of the uvula away from the side of the infection.[4]

Infections arise from tonsillitis. Diagnosis of a peritonsillar infection is often based on clinical presentation and careful examination of the oropharynx. It is important to distinguish cellulitis from a drainable abscess, which can be accomplished by attempting intraoral needle aspiration in cooperative patients or by using intraoral ultrasound. A contrast enhanced computed tomography (CECT) scan is required when attempts fail to obtain an aspirate, in the presence of trismus, in patients who do not improve with initial antibiotic therapy. Because of a higher recurrence rate, adults with peritonsillar infections generally should be treated subsequently with tonsillectomy.

Submandibular Space

It is composed of two potential spaces that span from the mucosal covering of the floor of the mouth down to the superficial layer of deep cervical fascia as it encloses the space between the mandible and the hyoid bone. The mylohyoid muscle traverses the space horizontally and divides it into a supramylohyoid compartment, also known as the anatomically correct submandibular or submaxillary space. The term "submandibular" will henceforth refer to the combined inframylohyoid and supramylohyoid compartments. These two compartments communicate freely along the posterior aspect of the mylohyoid muscle,[4] and infections have been noted to spread to the parapharyngeal space posteriorly and the anterior visceral space inferiorly.[2] The roots of the second and third mandibular molars lie below the attachment of the mylohyoid to the mandible and posterior dental infections can spread directly into the inframylohyoid compartments.

In contrast, the remaining mandibular dental roots lie above the mylohyoid line, and more anterior dental infections spread directly into the submylohyoid compartment. Other sources of infection include sialadentitis, suppurative lymphadenitis, oral trauma and upper respiratory infections. Aspirates from submandibular space infections reveal a prevalence of odontogenic pathogens, including aerobic *Streptococcus viridians* and staphylococci and anaerobic *Prevotella* and *Peptostreptococcus species.*[2]

The supramylohyoid compartment (sublingual space) contains loose areolar tissue, the sublingual glands, the submandibular (Wharton's) duct, geniohyoid muscles and the lingual and hypoglossal nerves. Supramylohyoid infections often present with induration, swelling and tenderness in the floor of the mouth that often begins laterally. Protrusion and elevation of the tongue can occur as the swelling proceeds medially.

The inframylohyoid compartment (submaxillary space) contains the anterior belly of the digastric muscles, submandibular glands and lymph nodes. The "mental space" refers to the portion of the inframylohyoid compartment confined between the anterior bellies of the digastric muscles. Inframylohyoid infections cause induration, swelling and tenderness below the mandible and can progress to elevation and protrusion of the tongue. Infection within this compartment requires an extraoral surgical approach.

Ludwig's Angina

Ludwig's angina is diagnosed clinically based on the classic description of the "rapidly spreading, firmly indurated cellulitis that originates intraorally and involves (supramylohyoid and inframylohyoid compartments) bilaterally, but without abscess or lymphadenopathy," resulting in rapidly progressing upper airway progression,[1] most cases are of odontogenic origin; less common include peritonsillar or parapharyngeal abscesses, epiglottitis and penetrating injuries to the floor of the mouth. Diabetics with impaired immune function are at increased risk of developing Ludwig's angina secondary to submandibular space infections.[2] Swelling within the enclosed submandibular space displaces the tongue superiorly and posteriorly and causes odynophagia, dysphagia and drooling. Tongue protrusion can potentially culminate in rapidly progressive airway obstruction and asphyxiation if the airway is not urgently addressed. Fiberoptic nasotracheal intubation may afford the best initial approach to airway management and should be attempted with the patient sitting up or in semi-Fowler position, rather than supine. Tracheotomy is the standard approach in Ludwig's angina patients who fail intubations.

The definitive treatment for Ludwig's angina involves early airway protection and a combination of broad-spectrum antibiotics and surgical decompression of a firmly indurated submandibular space. Ludwig's angina may lead to complications such as airway compromise, osteomyelitis of the mandible, pleural effusion, empyema and infection of carotid sheath structures.

Parapharyngeal Space

This is also known as the lateral parapharyngeal or pharyngomaxillary space, takes the form of an inverted pyramid extending from the base of the skull down to the hyoid bone. It lies between the visceral divisions of the middle layer of deep cervical fascia medially and the superficial layer of deep cervical fascia covering the pterygoid muscles and parotid gland laterally. The space is divided into two compartments by the styloid process and the stylohyoid, stylopharyngeus and styloglossus muscles. The prestyloid compartment lies anteriorly and contains the internal maxillary artery, maxillary nerve and adipose tissue, and the poststyloid compartment lies posteriorly and includes the neurovascular contents of the carotid sheath (carotid artery, internal jugular vein, cervical sympathetic chain and cranial nerves IX, X, XI and XII).[4]

Parapharyngeal infections have many sources because of the sheer number of neighboring deep neck compartments, which include the submandibular, retropharyngeal, parotid and masticator spaces. Causes include pharyngitis, tonsillitis, otitis, mastoiditis, parotitis and cervical lymphadenitis. Infection of the prestyloid compartment often presents clinically with fever, chills, neck pain, trismus and anteromedial displacement of the ipsilateral palatine tonsil. Infection of the poststyloid compartment has been known to cause little or no pain, trismus, or obvious swelling; however, involvement of the carotid sheath contents can lead to complications such as septicemia, Lemierre's syndrome; an infective internal jugular vein thrombosis (IJVT), or, carotid artery aneurysm or rupture, ipsilateral Horner's syndrome and cranial nerve IX through XII palsies.

The management of parapharyngeal space infections must begin with appropriate image to determine if an abscess is present, the extent of its spread and its proximity and relation to the carotid sheath contents. CECT of the head and neck, in combination with careful physical examination, have been shown to differentiate deep neck abscess from cellulitis most accurately. Infections involving the poststyloid compartment, but not the prestyloid compartment, were much more frequent in children and were likely the result of acute cervical lymphadenitis, a relatively benign condition that should respond well to an initial 48 hours of intravenous antibiotics. On the other hand, infections involving the prestyloid compartment were common to all ages and were principally a result of dental and pharyngeal infections. Prestyloid infections must be differentiated from poststyloid cervical lymphadenitis and that abscesses within the prestyloid compartment require prompt surgical drainage to avoid complications from the rapid spread of pus into adjacent deep neck spaces.

Surgical access of the parapharyngeal space by way of an external surgical approach, with an incision along the anterior-superior border of the SCM muscle to gain adequate exposure and avoid injuring the carotid sheath contents. Most recently, however, CECT has been used to identify accurately the parapharyngeal abscesses contained within the prestyloid compartment (anterior and medial to the carotid sheath) and has allowed for a less invasive transoral drainage approach to prestyloid infections. CECT scans often reveal a bulge of the ipsilateral pharyngeal wall and tonsil when an abscess involves the prestyloid compartment of the parapharyngeal space and that the bulge can serve as a landmark to guide intraoral incision and drainage in the pediatric population. Abscesses that spread into adjacent deep neck spaces and those that involving the poststyloid compartment require an external cervical approach to incision and drainage.

Masticator/Temporal Space

This lies between the medial pterygoid muscle and the more lateral masseter muscle and is enclosed by the divisions of the superficial layer of deep cervical fascia that envelop these muscles. It extends back to the posterior aspect of the mandible and superiorly as the temporal space, to surround the temporalis muscle deep to the temporalis fascia. Its contents include the temporalis muscle, the ramus of the mandible divisions of the mandibular nerve (V3), and the internal maxillary artery. Most infections originate from the posterior mandibular molars; less common sources include trauma and surgery. Patients often present severe trismus, sore throat, dysphagia, pain surrounding the ramus of the mandible and preauricular or mandibular swelling. More extensive infections can cause swelling of the entire side of the face and involvement of the orbit may lead to proptosis, optic neuritis and cranial nerve VI palsy. The surgical approach depends on the location of the abscess in relation to the mandible. An intraoral approach at the retromolar trigone is appropriate for draining abscesses medial to the ramus of the mandible and an extraoral approach along the inferior border of the mandible is used for draining abscesses lateral to the mandibular ramus. An incision through the temporalis fascia along the hairline is necessary to drain abscesses that spread superiorly and surround the temporalis muscle within the temporal space.[1,4]

Buccal Space

This lies between the buccopharyngeal fascia overlying the buccinator muscle medially and the skin of the cheek laterally and is limited inferiorly by the border of the mandible and posteriorly by the pterygomandibular raphe. It contains the buccal fat pad, the parotid duct and the facial artery. Most buccal face infections are odontogenic in origin and present with a warm and tender swelling within the cheek and minimal systemic symptoms. Trismus may be present if the infection spreads posteriorly to involve the masseter muscle.[1,4]

Parotid Space

This exists within the capsule that is formed by the superficial layer of deep cervical fascia as it envelops the parotid gland. The fascia on the medial aspect of the gland is thin and provides little resistance to the spread of parotid space infections into the adjacent parapharyngeal space. In addition to the parotid gland, the space also contains the facial nerve, external carotid artery, retromandibular vein, auriculotemporal nerve, superficial temporal artery and lymph nodes. Infections often result from parotid duct obstruction or suppurative lymphadenitis and occasionally originate from odontogenic infections of the mandibular molars that traverse the masticator space. Patients usually present with severe pain and swelling at the angle of the mandible, but little or no trismus unless the masticator space is sufficiently involved. Systematic symptoms such as fever and chills may accompany the spread of infection into the parapharyngeal space and other deep neck spaces. An external, parotidectomy-like approach is used to drain a parotid space abscess and blunt dissection, either superior or inferior to the posterior belly of the digastric muscle, allows concurrent drainage of the parapharyngeal space when it is involved.[1,4]

Spaces that Involve the Entire Length of the Neck

Retropharyngeal Space

The retropharyngeal space lies between the visceral (buccopharyngeal) fascia covering the posterior pharynx and esophagus and the alar fascia, a division of the deep layer of deep cervical fascia and occupies the space posterior to the pharynx and esophagus. It extends from the base of skull down into the mediastinum, where the visceral and alar fascia fuse at the level of the second thoracic vertebra. Laterally, it is bounded by the carotid sheaths. The retropharyngeal space is fused down the midline and contains two chains of lymph nodes extending down each side. Retropharyngeal abscesses are unilateral because of the midline fusion and are primarily seen early in childhood. Upper respiratory infections cause most retropharyngeal disease in children because these lymph nodes receive drainage from the nose, sinuses and pharynx. Retropharyngeal infection is also seen following trauma to the posterior pharynx or as an extension from an adjacent parapharyngeal space infection.[4] Cultures of retropharyngeal aspirates are generally polymicrobial and contain common oropharyngeal flora such as *S. viridians*.

Children with retropharyngeal infection often present with neck pain, neck swelling, fever, irritability, dysphagia, excessive drooling and dyspnea or noisy breathing suggestive of upper airway compromise.[2,4] Adults tend to present with neck pain, fever, anorexia, nasal obstruction, snoring and dyspnea.[1] Careful oropharyngeal examination often reveals unilateral bulging of the posterior pharynx, which is localized in retropharyngeal lymphadenitis and may extend the length of the pharynx when cellulitis or an abscess is present. In the absence of acute distress, CECT of the head and neck can be used to confirm the diagnosis and evaluate for spread of infection into the adjacent deep neck spaces.[4]

The most feared complications are airway obstruction and rupture of an abscess with subsequent aspiration of pus. Patients who have signs of airway compromise should be taken immediately to the operating room before being examined. With the patient in the head-down Trendelenburg's position and intubated along the opposite side of the pharynx from the swelling, needle aspiration should precede intraoral incision and drainage, to obtain specimens for culture and sensitivity and to minimize any risk of the patient aspirating pus during the procedure. Spread of the infection into the parapharyngeal space may necessitate an external cervical approach to incision and drainage if the involvement is not confirmed to the prestyloid compartment medial to the great vessels.[4]

Danger Space

The danger space lies posterior to the retropharyngeal space between the alar and prevertebral fascias, the two divisions of the deep layer of deep cervical fascia and extends from the skull base down into the posterior mediastinum to the level of the diaphragm. Infections indirectly result from the spread of retropharyngeal, parapharyngeal and prevertebral space abscesses. The "danger" lies in the tendency for infections to spread inferiorly through the space and into the thorax because the loose areolar contents offer little resistance, resulting in complications such as mediastinitis, empyema and sepsis. Danger space infections initially present in the same way as retropharyngeal infections and CECT is necessary to differentiate between them.[1]

Prevertebral Space

This space is a potential space between the prevertebral fascia and the underlying vertebral bodies and deep cervical musculature. It extends down the entire length of the vertebral column to the coccyx. However, dense fibrous attachments between the prevertebral fascia and deep cervical muscles tend to contain prevertebral infections and help prevent longitudinal spread. Sources of infection include trauma to the posterior pharynx and secondary spread from Pot's abscesses and retropharyngeal and danger space infections. Patients often present with midline bulge in posterior pharynx. Complications include osteomyelitis and spinal instability, which require a prolonged course of antibiotics. Once identified with CECT, prevertebral space abscesses should be drained using an external cervical approach rather than an intraoral approach, which can lead to a persistent draining fistula in the posterior pharynx.[4]

Carotid Space

The carotid (visceral vascular) space lies within the cervical sheath and houses the carotid artery, internal jugular vein, cervical sympathetic chain and cranial nerves IX, X, XI and XII. It is similar to the prevertebral space, in that, it contains little areolar tissue and thus is somewhat resistant to the longitudinal spread of infection.

However, "Lincoln's highway" suggests, the carotid sheath receives contributions from all three nerves of deep cervical fascia, extends from the base of skull into the mediastinum and can potentially serve as a highway for infectious spread originating in any deep neck space. In addition to secondary spread from adjacent deep neck spaces, direct inoculation into the neck in intravenous drug abusers and iatrogenic causes such as central venous catheterization can lead to carotid space infections. Patients often present with stiffness and ipsilateral swelling of the neck, fever, chills, ipsilateral Horner's syndrome, vocal cord paralysis and other complication-related findings. IJVT can issue intermittent spiking fevers, and carotid artery rupture may be preceded by sentinel blebs from the ear, nose or mouth. An external cervical approach is used for incision and drainage of the carotid space.[1,4]

Space Below the Level of the Hyoid Bone

Anterior Visceral Space

This is the only deep neck space limited below the hyoid bone. It is bounded by the visceral division of the middle layer of deep cervical fascia and lies between the infrahyoid strap muscles and the esophagus. It contains the thyroid gland, the trachea and the anterior wall of the esophagus and extends from the thyroid cartilage down into the superior mediastinum overlying the aortic arch and fibrous pericardium. The anterior visceral space lies anterior and the retropharyngeal space lies posterior to the esophagus.[4]

Infections of the anterior visceral space often originate from traumatic perforation of the anterior esophageal wall and, less commonly, from neck trauma or thyroiditis. They often present with neck swelling, sore throat, dysphagia, hoarseness and dyspnea because of pharyngeal, laryngeal and supraglottic edema, which can potentially progress to airway compromise. In addition, the perforation of visceral contents may cause crepitation of the anterior neck, mediastinitis and pneumothorax.[4] Abscesses in the anterior visceral space require an external cervical approach to incision and drainage.[4]

DIAGNOSING DEEP NECK INFECTION

History, physical examination, laboratory work and diagnostic imaging, each provides important clues when assessing a patient for DNI. Initial evaluation of the airway is the first priority and any signs of respiratory distress or impending airway compromise should be immediately and aggressively managed. Potential sources of the infection such as any recent illness, dental caries or procedures, trauma to the head and neck or intravenous drug use should be uncovered. Risk factors including diabetic mellitus, HIV infection, steroid therapy, chemotherapy and other sources of immune dysfunction should be identified early and appropriately managed to minimize potential complications.

Other common symptoms were space specific and included dysphagia, trismus, dysphonia, otalgia and dyspnea. In the pediatric population, fever, neck mass and neck stiffness were almost prevalent, followed by sore throat, poor oral intake, drooling and lymphadenopathy.[2] Infants less than 9 months old most often present with a neck mass or swelling, lymphadenopathy, fever, rhinorrhea, poor oral intake and cough.[2]

HIV screening in adults; blood cultures and appropriate cultures of aspirates obtained before antibiotics are instituted, if possible. Culture results are most accurate when obtained with needle aspiration and specimens for anaerobic cultures should be placed immediately into an oxygen-free container. In addition to aerobic and anaerobic cultures, fungal and acid-fast cultures are recommended for immunocompromised patients.[4] Negative cultures, despite the finding of organisms on gram stain, may suggest an anaerobic infection. Additional testing for atypical causes of DNI, such as *Bartonella henselae* (cat scratch disease), *Mycobacterium*, or fungal infection, may be appropriate when cultures are negative.[2]

Diagnostic Imaging

Contrast enhanced computed tomography (CECT) has made an important contribution in characterizing the nature of a deep neck lesion. It is important in planning the surgical approach and is the current standard of care when managing a suspected DNI.[3] In addition, CECT has been shown to identify impending airway complications before they present clinically. Neck swelling that extends to the suprasternal notch may indicate involvement of the mediastinum and CECT should include the chest in such cases. Serial CT scanning may be useful in monitoring patients who have mediastinitis. Chest radiograph is useful when screening for complications such as mediastinitis, pneumonia and pleural effusion. However, CECT is superior for evaluating cellulitis or abscess within the mediastinum. Lateral neck radiographs have been used to screen for retropharyngeal and parapharyngeal abscesses. Dental radiographs, such as the panorex oral view, are useful in identifying odontogenic sources of infection.[1]

Ultrasound is more accurate than CECT in differentiating a drainable abscess from cellulitis.[4] The ultrasound should be used to supplement CECT or MRI in cases when the presence of a deep neck abscess is uncertain and to guide diagnostic and therapeutic needle or catheter aspiration of superficial, uniloculated fluid collections when imminent airway compromise is not evident.[4] Magnetic resonance angiography (MRA) is especially useful in evaluating vascular complications, such as IJVT and carotid artery aneurysm or rupture.

Airway Management

Acute airway obstruction is one of the most frequent and deadly complications of DNI. It is most often encountered in cases with multiple space involvement,

Ludwig's angina, or retropharyngeal, parapharyngeal, or anterior visceral space abscesses. Tracheotomy under local anesthesia, has been shown to be safe and effective and is considered by some to be the standard of care for managing airway compromise in DNI patients. Other methods of airway management include endotracheal intubation, fiberoptic nasotracheal intubation and cricothyrotomy. Each has advantages and disadvantages that must be carefully considered when selecting the safest and most appropriate method.

Careful monitoring of airway is the first priority. Indications for aggressive airway management include signs of respiratory distress (dyspnea, stridor, retractions) or impending airway compromise as noted on physical examination or diagnostic imaging (severe swelling within pharynx, upward displacement of the tongue airway edema or airway compression by an abscess). In advanced cases of DNI, placing the patient in the supine position may precipitate complete airway obstruction, which is important to consider when sedating a supine patient or sending them for an MRI without first securing his or her airway.[3,4] Routine use of intravenous steroids in patients who have impending airway obstruction can minimize swelling and reduce the need for aggressive airway intervention.[3] However, systemic steroids have hyperglycemic effects and should be avoided in patients who have diabetes mellitus or poor glucose control.

Endotracheal intubation may be attempted before tracheotomy in most patients who have DNL. It is often made difficult by distorted airway anatomy, immobility of the soft tissues or trismus that limits access to the mouth. Extreme care should be taken in the presence of pharyngeal wall abscess because of the risk of rupture and subsequent aspiration of pus. Trismuses may be overcome with the use of general anesthesia. However, in most advanced cases, general anesthesia is dangerous and can precipitate complete airway obstruction that necessitates an emergency tracheotomy.[3,4] Unplanned extubation is the most common complication of endotracheal intubation. Both planned and unplanned extubation risk airway loss secondary to worsening laryngeal edema and subsequent inability to reintubate, which is an avoidable source of mortality.

Fiberoptic nasotracheal intubation, is useful in patients who have severe trismus but whose airways are otherwise uncompromised.[2] Tracheotomy under local anesthesia is indicated for severe or impending airway obstruction when trismus or massive soft tissue edema precludes endotracheal intubation or when repeated attempts at intubation have failed.[4] Separate incisions should be used for tracheotomy and drainage procedures of the anterior neck to avoid infectious spread into the mediastinum. Tracheotomy should be avoided if possible when the pretracheal or anterior visceral space is involved in the infection. Cricothyrotomy, or emergency tracheotomy, can provide urgent airway access when complete loss of the airway necessitates immediate surgical intervention. Passage of the cricothyrotomy tube may cause trauma to the posterior wall of the trachea and subglottic stenosis is a potential complication. Cricothyrotomy should be converted to a standard tracheotomy within 24 to 48 hours.

Microbiology

Cultures of aspirates from deep neck space abscesses are commonly polymicrobial and reflect the oropharyngeal flora and odontogenic nature of these infections. Frequently isolated aerobes include *S. viridians*, *Klebsiella pneumonae*, and *S. aureus*, and less frequently, *Streptococcus pneumonia*, *Streptococcus pyogenes*, *Neisseria* species, and *Haemophilus influenzae*. Common anaerobic isolates include *Peptostreptococcus*, *Bacteroides fragilis*, pigmented *Prevotella* and *Porphyromonas* species, *Fusobacterium* species, and *Eikenella corrodens*. Anaerobic bacteria are increasingly penicillin-resistant because of production of beta-lactase, which is released into the infection and has a protective effect for nearby penicillin-sensitive species. *E. corrodens*, an anaerobe frequently isolated in children and intravenous drug abusers, is universally resistant to clindamycin and metronidazole, but is sensitive to penicillin and aminoglycosides. In addition, methicillin-resistant *S. aureus* (MRSA), once considered a nosocomial infection as been seen with increasing prevalence as a community acquired cause of DNI in intravenous drug abusers, immunocompromised patients, infants and young children.

The MRSA is an emerging pathogen in necrotizing fasciitis and descending mediastinitis. *K. pneumonia* is, consistently, the most common cause of DNI in patients who have poorly controlled diabetes mellitus.

Empiric Antibiotic Coverage

Every patient who has a DNI should be given initial empiric antibiotic therapy until culture and sensitivity results are available. Empiric antibiotic therapy should be effective against the aerobic and anaerobic bacteria that are commonly involved, and, once available, the results of the culture and sensitivity test can allow for tailoring of adequate antibiotic therapy. Either penicillin in combination with a β-lactamase-resistant inhibitor (such as amoxicillin or ticarcillin with clavulanic acid) or a β-lactamase-resistant antibiotic (such as cefoxitin, cefuroxime, imipenem or meropenem) in combination with a drug that is highly effective against most anaerobes (such as clindamycin or metronidazole) is recommended for optimal empiric coverage.[3] Vancomycin should be considered for empiric therapy in intravenous drug abusers at risk for infection with MRSA[1] and in patients who have profound neutropenia or immune dysfunction. Ceftriaxone and clindamycin can be used as empiric therapy against community-acquired MRSA in young children. The addition of gentamicin for effective gram-negative coverage against *K. pneumonia*, which is resistant to clindamycin, is highly recommended for diabetic patients. However, renal function should be closely monitored. Parental antibiotic therapy should be continued until the patient has been afebrile for at least 48 hours, followed by oral therapy using amoxicillin with clavulanic acid, clindamycin, ciprofloxacin, trimethoprim-sulfamethoxazole or metronidazole.[1]

Conservative Medical Management

Surgical drainage is the classical approach to any DNI with suspected abscess formation and is felt by many investigators to be the first-line treatment in these cases.[2] Recent studies, however, are beginning to show that, in selected cases, an uncomplicated deep neck abscess or cellulitis can be effectively treated with antibiotics and careful monitoring, without surgical drainage. The use of steroids along with antibiotic treatment may reduce the need for surgical intervention by minimizing airway edema, inflammation and the progression of cellulitis into an abscess.[2] However, conservative management may not be effective for diabetic patients who have demonstrated a lack of response to that treatment.[3] Aspiration of an abscess for culture and sensitivity is recommended for immunocompromised patients and anyone at risk for infection with an unusual or atypical pathogen.[4]

Surgical Intervention

Surgical intervention remains the mainstay of treatment for more complicated or severe cases of DNI. Indications for surgery include airway compromise, critical condition, septicemia, complications, descending infection, diabetes mellitus, or no clinical improvement within 48 hours of the initiation of parenteral antibiotics.[1,4] In addition, abscesses greater than 3 cm in diameter that involve the prevertebral, anterior visceral, or carotid spaces, or that involve more than two spaces, should be surgically drained.[2] Surgical drainage can be performed in several ways, including simple intraoral or extraoral incision and drainage for superficial abscesses, a more extensive external cervical approach for deeper and more complicated infections, and minimally invasive techniques such as image guided needle aspiration and indwelling catheter placement.

Fluid resuscitation before surgery is important in DNI patients because they frequently present in a dehydrated state.[1] The external cervical approach is most often used when draining the anterior visceral, submandibular, parapharyngeal, prevertebral and carotid spaces and for complicated retropharyngeal abscesses that cannot be fully drained using an intraoral approach.[4] Wide exposure of the infected tissue is important, as in debridement of any necrotic tissue that is present. Wounds requiring extensive debridement should be left opened and packed with antimicrobial dressings to allow for frequent inspection. Wounds with less necrosis can be closed at surgery with active suction drainage. In cases involving descending infections, cervical drainage is sufficient as long as the infection remains above the carina. Transthoracic drainage is necessary when infection spreads below the carina.[1]

Minimally invasive techniques have been used more recently for well-defined, unilocular abscesses in patients who do not have airway compromise. Ultrasound guidance is appropriate for locating and draining abscesses accessible through the skin and CT guidance is helpful when attempting needle aspiration of a deep, difficult to access collection of fluid. Needle aspiration and catheter placement offer the advantages of a small point of entry, quick healing time, little or no scar formation and less risk of contaminating the surrounding deep neck spaces while draining pus.

COMPLICATIONS

Mediastinitis results from downward extension of an infection that involves the spaces that extend the length of the neck or the anterior visceral space. The causative organism varies depending on the origin of the infection; most cases are polymicrobial and involve both aerobes and anaerobes.[2]

Afflicted patients will frequently complain of increasing chest pain or dyspnea and chest radiography or CECT may demonstrate a widened mediastinum of pneumomediastinum.[2] Transthoracic drainage is necessary when the infection spreads below the carina.

Lemierre's syndrome, or suppurative thrombophlebitis of the internal jugular vein, results from extension of the infection into the carotid space. Pathognomonic findings include swelling and tenderness at the angle of the jaw and along the SCM muscle, along with signs of sepsis (spiking fever, chills) and evidence of pulmonary emboli.[2] IJVT may be detected using high, resolution ultrasound, CEC, or MRI/MRA. Treatment involves prolonged antimicrobial therapy directed by culture and sensitivity results and anticoagulation is currently recommended for 3 months when thrombus progression or septic emboli are present. Most cases resolve with antibiotic and anticoagulation therapy and do not require surgical ligation and resection of the internal jugular vein. Fibrinolytic agents may be used if IJVT is recognized within 4 days of onset, but they carry a higher risk of hemorrhage than anticoagulation. Endovascular stenting is another option for patients available to tolerate long-term anticoagulation and superior vena cava filters have reportedly been used in selected cases.[2]

Carotid artery aneurysm or rupture maybe present with a pulsatile neck mass and often results in four cardinal signs:

- Recurrent sentinel hemorrhages from the pharynx or ear
- Protracted clinical course (7 to 14 days)
- Hematoma of the surrounding neck tissues
- Hemodynamic collapse.

Early recognition and surgical intervention of the common carotid artery is essential. Necrotizing cervical fasciitis is a fulminant infection that spreads along fascial planes and causes necrosis of connective tissue. The pathogens involved are usually polymicrobial and odontogenic and they include *S. pyogenes, Clostridium perfringens* and mixed aerobes and anaerobes. Patients who have necrotizing fasciitis are acutely ill with high fever, and the skin overlying the necrosis may be tender, edematous and erythematous, with indistinct transition to normal skin. Soft tissue crepitation due to infection with gas-producing organisms may be present and, in more advanced cases, the skin becomes pale, aesthetic and dusky with blistering and sloughing.[1] CECT may demonstrate diffuse cellulitis with infiltration of the skin and the subcutaneous tissues and myositis, compartmental fluid and gas accumulations.[2] Managing necrotizing fasciitis is best accomplished in an ICU and frequent surgical debridement of any devitalized tissue. The wound should be left open and packed with antimicrobial dressings until the infection has subsided. Hyperbaric oxygen is useful as an adjunctive treatment in hemodynamically stable patients.

Aspiration pneumonia, lung abscess, empyema and even asphyxiation may result when an abscess ruptures into the larynx or trachea and purulent drainage is subsequently aspirated. Horner's syndrome and cranial nerve IX and XII palsies result from infections that invade the carotid space. Osteomyelitis can involve the mandible or cranial vertebral bodies, and can lead to vertebral subluxation.[4] Sepsis is often cited as a direct cause of mortality in DNI studies.

REFERENCES

1. Weed HG, Forest LA. Deep neck infection. In: Cummings CW, Flint PW, Harker LA, et al. (Ed). Otolaryngology: Head and Neck Surgery, 4th edition. Philadelphia: Elsevier Mosby; 2005;3:2515-24.
2. Vieria F, Allen SM, Stocks RMS, Thompson JW. Deep neck infection. In: Dornhoffer JL, Chandra RK. (Ed). Otolaryngologic Clinics of North America, Philadelphia: WB Saunders Company; 2008;41(3):459-81.
3. Boscolo-Rizzo P, et al. Conservative management of deep neck abscesses in adults: The importance of CECT findings. Otolaryngol Head & Neck Surg. 2006;135(6):894-9.
4. Yellon RF. Head and neck space infections. In: Bluestone CD, Casselbrat ML, Stool SE, et al. (Ed). Pediatric Otolaryngology, 4th edition. Philadelphia: Saunders; 2003;2:1681-701.

CHAPTER

4 Tracheostomy

INTRODUCTION

Establishing and maintaining patent upper airway is the first and most vital step in the basic life support and maintenance, and artificial airway is the most fundamental aspect of such support. The ability to quickly assess the situation, plan the approach and intervene by successfully securing an airway is essential.

The goal of difficult airway management is rapid control and correction of an impending airway obstruction.[1] Tracheostomy is an important procedure in difficult airway management. Modern approaches to open tracheostomy still draw on classic description of Chevalier Jackson (Figure 4.1).

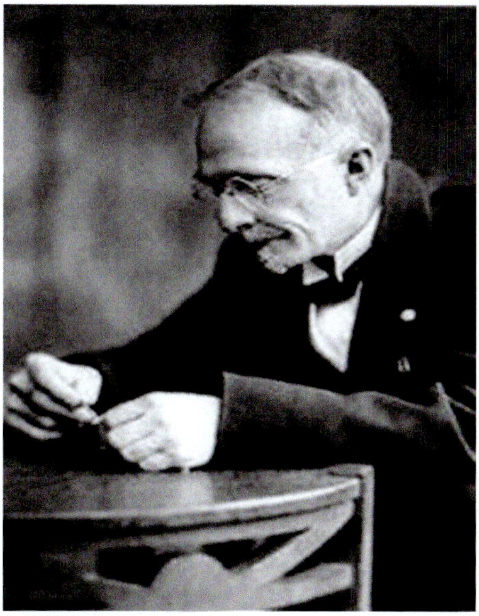

Figure 4.1 Chevalier Jackson (Pioneer for modern tracheostomy)

"Tracheostomy" is the term used to describe the surgical opening of trachea. Although "Tracheostomy" is used to describe the creation of stoma at skin surface, which leads to trachea.

Tracheostomy is a common procedure in the intensive care unit and approximately 13% of ICU patients will have a tracheostomy at one point of time.[2] The growth of nasotracheal or orotracheal intubation or percutaneous tracheostomy, particularly later in the past 10 years has meant that the surgical management of upper airway obstruction is no longer the exclusive province of otolaryngologist.

HISTORICAL PERSPECTIVE

In the history of tracheostomy, it was divided into FIVE phases:

- **Period of Legends** (2000 BC–1546 AD)

  In this period, tracheostomy was very common and used for relieving upper airway obstruction. The pros and cons of the procedure are analyzed during this period. In spite of criticizations from various legends like Hippocrates, Caelius Aurelianus, Aretaeus, etc., it was advocated by experts like Asclepiades, Antyllus, Paulus von Aegina
- **Period of Fear** (1546–1833 AD)

  Tracheostomy was done by few during this phase. There was widespread stigma on performing the procedure fearing its complications. The first documented case of a successful tracheostomy, the first pediatric tracheostomy and the name "TRACHEOSTOMY" were given during this period (Figure 4.2)

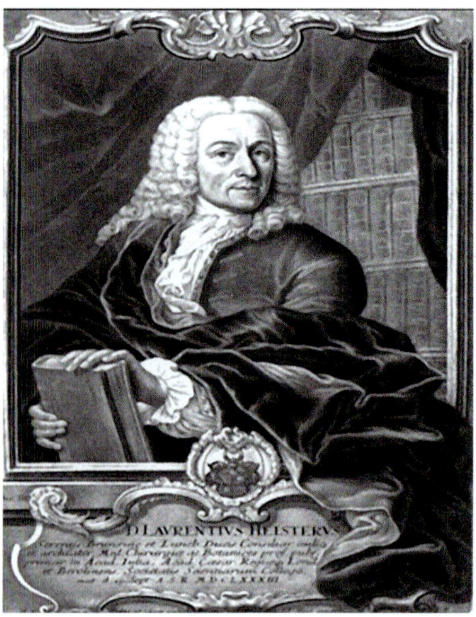

Figure 4.2 Lorenz Heister (Man who coined the term "Tracheostomy")

- **Period of Drama** (1833–1932 AD)

  This period starts with Trousseau's report of 200 cases in the therapy of diphtheria in 1833. Tracheostomy became a highly dramatized operation for asphyxia and acute respiratory obstruction and also the importance of post-operative care for tracheostomy was stressed
- **Period of Enthusiasm** (1932–1965 AD)

  In this time, the adage—"If you think Tracheostomy—do it", became popular. Its use in poliomyelitis was known and it was also recommended for a variety of mixed illnesses
- **Period of Rationalization** (1965 AD–present)

  Complications, indications and interrelation with endotracheal intubation are clearly defined during this phase. The development of synthetic materials and low pressure/high volume cuffs have improved the tracheostomy tubes and reduced the complication rate of the procedure. The advent of *percutaneous tracheostomy* further revolutionized the procedure.

Tracheostomy has a long and colorful history. The oldest evidence for tracheostomy comes from sacred Hindu book, The Rigveda, from approximately 2000 BC. It has been mentioned in the book as "... The bountiful one who, without a ligature, can cause the windpipe to reunite when the cervical cartilages are cut across ...". It also describes about healing of a tracheostomy incision.

It was described by Homer in his quotes and in the review of history of tracheostomy by Frost, that in around 1000 BC it was performed by Alexander—The Great, as an aid to save a choking soldier with his sword (Figure 4.3).

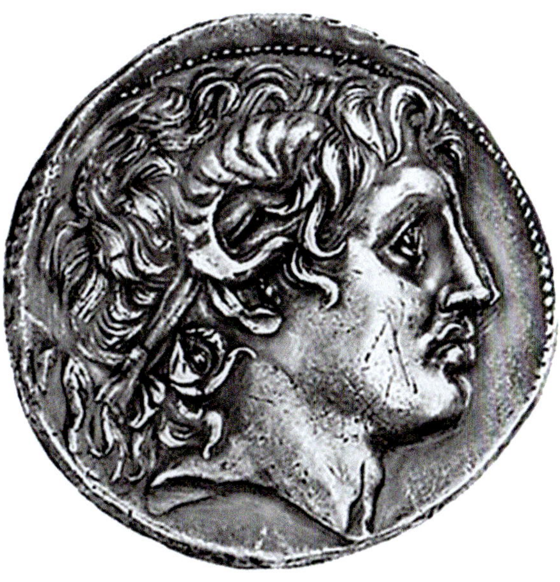

Figure 4.3 Alexander—The Great (who allegedly did tracheostomy to a choking soldier)

Asclepiades of Bithynia–124 BC is credited for describing tracheostomy incision for some nonspecific inflammatory condition of larynx, floor of the mouth.

Galen and Aretaeus wrote about the procedure and attribute its performance to Ascepiades, a physician of second century AD. After Galen's description of laryngeal anatomy, the practice of performing the procedure increased.

In 2nd century AD, Tracheostomy technique was further defined by Antyllas (625–690 AD), a greek surgeon who advised that trachea should be divided at the III and IV ring using a transverse incision, to minimize cartilage damage.

In 7th century AD, Paul of Aegina recorded that physician could be aware that if the airway is entered, a rush of air would be heard and loss of patient's voice would be noted.

The first documented case of successful tracheostomy was done by Antonio Musa Brassavola in 1546 (Figure 4.4).

Sanctorius (1561–1636 AD) is believed to be the first to use a trocar and cannula in the operation and he recommended leaving the cannula in place for 3 days, following the operation.

Marco Aurelio Severino (1580–1656 AD) used the Tracheostomy to save multiple lives during the 1610 diphtheria epidemic in Naples. He also developed his own version of a trocar.

The first book on tracheostomy was written by a French surgeon Nicholas Habicot (1550–1624 AD). In 1620, he described four successful tracheostomies. One of these, performed on an 14-year-old boy, was possibly the first successful

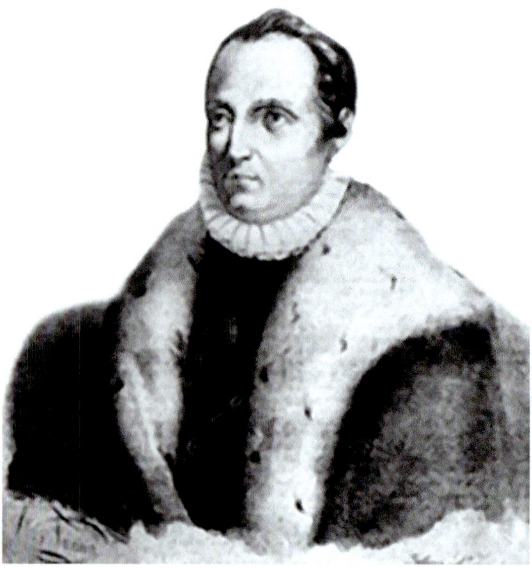

Figure 4.4 Antonio Musa Brassavola (did first documented successful tracheostomy)

pediatric tracheostomy and he was the first to record a case of tracheostomy for the removal of a foreign body by using curved metal tube. He also performed a series of four tracheostomies for obstructing foreign bodies.

The term Tracheostomy was actually coined by Lorenz Heister in 1718 (Figure 4.2). It was previously called as laryngotomy or bronchotomy.

George Martine (1702–1743 AD), the earliest known British tracheostomist suggested use of an inner cannula in the tracheostomy tube in 1730.

In 1799, George Washington at Mount Vernon, Virginia, died of an upper airway obstruction probably due to acute epiglottitis or an inflammatory Quinsy.

In 1805, Viq d'Azur described cricothyrotomy.

Pierre Bretonneau (1778–1862 AD), published report of a successful tracheostomy in a 5-year-old girl with diphtheria in 1825.

In 1833, Trousseau reported survival of 50 out of 200 tracheostomies in children with diphtheria and also stressed techniques for postoperative care for the first time (Figure 4.5).

In 1909, Chevalier Jackson, described the standard surgical tracheostomy (in which dissection of the strap muscles was followed by controlled entry into the trachea). He also described that two chief preventable sequelae of the procedure are death from improper routine surgical care and wrongly fitted tube and stenosis from a higher incision. He condemned the use of cough suppressants or narcotics, postoperatively.

In 1943, Galloway, reported the usefulness of the procedure for respiratory care of patients with poliomyelitis.

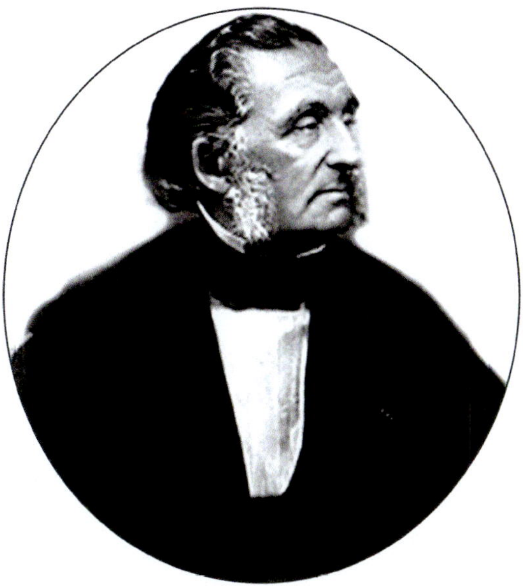

Figure 4.5 Armond Trousseau (emphasized postoperative care)

The vertical incision was introduced by Fabricius to reduce blood vessel injury and also to achieve greater exposure.

In 1955, Sheldon CH first attempted percutaneous tracheostomy with a slotted needle and a cutting trocar to create an opening in the trachea.

Toye and Weinstein developed percutaneous tracheostomy, influenced by the Seldinger technique in 1969—method of using a single-tapered dilator with a recessed cutting blade.

In 1965, A Berden introduced polyvinyl chloride tracheostomy tube.

In 1965, McDonald and Stocks described the use of intubations and respiratory support for neonatal patients.

In 1985, Ciaglia P discovered the technique known as percutaneous dilational tracheostomy and described the method via the Seldinger approach in 1989.

Schachner A developed the Rapitrach method of percutaneous tracheostomy by forcibly advancing a beveled metal conus over a wire in 1989.

In 1990, Griggs WM, presented guidewire dilating forceps method.

INDICATIONS

Tracheostomy is usually performed in case of upper airway obstruction (now it has become unusual after the advent of intubation), removal of secretions, in cases of prolonged ventilation and as part of a major surgery.

Upper Airway Obstruction

Cause may be inside or outside the larynx.

- Congenital[2]
    - Pierre Robin syndrome
    - Subglottic stenosis
    - Macroglossia
    - Treacher Collins syndrome
    - Goldenhar syndrome
    - Cystic hygroma
    - Choanal atresia
    - Supraglottic cyst
    - Congenital bilateral abductor palsy
    - Laryngeal web
    - Laryngomalacia
- Traumatic
    - External trauma
        - Maxillofacial injuries
        - Neck contusion
        - Laryngeal fractures

- Internal trauma:
    - Foreign bodies
    - Burns
    - Iatrogenic injuries
    - Prolonged intubation

In a study made by GT Schneider with 158 patients, early tracheostomy done in 43 patients had low incidence of ventilator associated pneumonia and less hospital stay compared to the late tracheostomy cases.[3]

- Infections
    - Epiglottitis
    - ALTB (acute laryngotracheobronchitis)
    - Cellulitis of neck (Ludwig's angina)
    - Retropharyngeal abscess
    - Diphtheria
- Tumors of the larynx
    - Papilloma
    - Hemangioma
    - Lymphangioma
    - Other carcinomas
- Neurogenic
    - Bilateral vocal cord paralysis.

Pulmonary Toilet and Protection of Airway

- Head injury
- Drug intoxication
- Encephalitis
- Degenerative lesions of spinal cord.

Recent Indication

- Sleep apnea syndrome
- Chronic obstructive pulmonary disease and emphysema
- Ondine's curse (primary alveolar hypoventilation syndrome)
- Home mechanical ventilation.[4]

In a study done by Argyro Amygdalou et al., on immediate postoperative effects of tracheostomy on pulmonary function, they found that there is significant decrease in pulmonary resistance and increase in pulmonary elastance after tracheostomy.[5]

SURGICAL ANATOMY

A breadth of understanding of the airway anatomy in relation to patient's age and underlying etiology are key to prepare for the subsequent intervention.

The cricoid cartilage is the only complete ring in the airway. The AP diameter of trachea is 24.33 mm in men and 19.19 mm in women and the mean lateral diameter is 24.33 mm and 18.51 mm respectively. The dimensions suggest that cricoid cartilage is approximately circular in adults. The distance between two vocal cords differs from person to person and can be assessed by direct laryngoscope prior to intubation.

Cricothyroid space is space between the cricoid and thyroid cartilages and when planning for cricothyroidotomy, two important anatomical features should be kept in mind. They are:

- Size of cricothyroid space:

  Vertically it is 9.61 mm in males and 7.85 mm in females. When the two cartilages are separated anteriorly, the cricothyroid space increases to 13.27 mm in males and 11.12 mm in females
- Size of the tube:

  Standard tracheostomy tube is different from that of airway configuration at cricothyroidotomy site and when inserted through a cricothyroidotomy site, the tracheostomy tube severely impinges the posterior tracheal wall, thereby traumatizing the tracheal mucosa.

Trachea is a cylindrical tube that extends inferiorly and posteriorly from the larynx into the thorax, where it bifurcates into the two main stem bronchi. The trachea consists of a series of C-shaped cartilages connected by connective tissue. The structure is supported on its anterior and lateral walls, while the posterior wall is membranous, overlying the esophagus closely. The length of the adult trachea is about 12 cm and its cross-sectional area is about 2.5 cm square. The trachea enters the thorax at approximately the level of the sixth tracheal cartilage. The trachea is lined with ciliated epithelium containing large number of mucus glands and goblet cells. The contraction of the transverse fibers of the smooth muscle in trachea can narrow the tracheal lumen and stabilize it.

The blood supply to the trachea in the neck is from branches of the inferior thyroid arteries and its venous drainage ends in the thyroid venous plexus. Its innervation is from two sources, the vagus with its recurrent branches and the sympathetic system.

One of the factors contributing to damage resulting from long-term intubation with a cuffed tube may be significant deformation of the trachea caused by a high pressure cuff. If the anteroposterior and lateral diameters could be identified prior to endotracheal intubation, an anatomically designed cuff might reduce damage inflicted during prolonged intubation. At present, no cost-effective technique exist to provide this information or to construct a tube to suit each individuals anatomy.[4]

TYPES OF TRACHEOSTOMY

According to Purpose

Temporary

Once the purpose is served, the tracheostomy is allowed to close.

Permanent

Tracheostomy tube remains in situ permanently, e.g. after laryngectomy.

According to Timing of Surgery

Elective Tracheostomy

Elective tracheostomy is feasible when airway obstruction is anticipated but not imminent or when planning for a procedure in head and neck that may cause upper airway swelling or obstruction.

Urgent Tracheostomy (Awake)

Indicated in patients with respiratory distress and needs immediate surgical intervention. Mostly done in ICU.

Emergent Tracheostomy (or Slash Trash)

Indicated in case of emergency airway distress. It is usually an indication of cricothyroidotomy and slash trash is performed when there is impossibility for cricothyroidotomy.[6]

According to the Level of Procedure

- High: Through the 2nd and 3rd tracheal rings
- Mid: Through the 3rd and 4th tracheal rings
- Low: Through the 4th and 5th tracheal rings.

EVALUATION

The severity or completeness of airway obstruction can be defined as:

- Complete obstruction—No detectable airflow in and out of the lungs
- Partial obstruction—Patient may be with stridor or respiratory difficulty
- Potential or Impending airway obstruction—Chance of developing airway obstruction due to known anatomical or physical abnormality.

If the situation is not urgent, a detailed history is obtained. The progression or regression and severity of symptoms should be noted. The history must also address difficulty with previous general anesthesia, sleep apnea or snoring, head and neck abnormalities and other coexisting diseases that might impair the airway.

In adults, the examination should be carefully done to note facial and neck masses and deformities, scars, quality of dentition, maxillary and mandibular position, pharyngeal structures and neck mobility.

In children, history regarding birth trauma and congenital abnormalities should be done. The history of an unexplained coughing episode is suggestive of a foreign body of the larynx, trachea or bronchi.

Anatomical difference between the adult and pediatric airway includes location of larynx in neck, increased airway collapsibility (which attributes to easy obstruction in younger patients), decreased functional pulmonary reserve and less developed accessory muscles of respiration.[6]

EFFECTS OF TRACHEOSTOMY

- Laryngeal bypass: Patients will be unable to cough or phonate
- Reduction in respiratory dead space
- Tendency for mucus collection in the redundant space between tracheal opening and larynx
- Loss of filtration of particulate matter and humidification of inspired air
- Increased risk of infection
- Problems with the inserted tracheostomy tube viz abrasions in the tracheal wall during neck movements.[2]

PROCEDURE

Anesthesia

It may be in general or with sedation in emergency situations, local anesthesia can be used (e.g. in ICU setup). Drugs that might depress the respiratory system should not be given in the preoperative period. Local anesthesia can be done with 1% lignocaine or procaine and 1:200,000 adrenaline. Before opening trachea, 0.5 mL of 4% lignocaine can be injected into the tracheal lumen to suppress cough during the procedure.

Positioning

Supine position with head extended to give prominence to the trachea and larynx.

Method

- Incision: Transverse incision, approximately 5 cm in length, just below the lower border of cricoid cartilage

- Subcutaneous fat, deep cervical fascia separated and flaps raised through blunt dissection of adjacent structures, until anterior jugular veins and infrahyoid muscles are exposed
- Separation of infrahyoid muscles done with blunt dissection
- Dividing of thyroid isthmus to be done with electrocautery or ligation
- Trachea entered by making a transverse incision over inter-cartilaginous ring of 2nd and 3rd tracheal cartilage. The incision can be extended and made into a circular opening. A flap of anterior wall of trachea can be raised and sutured to the skin margin of the incision, in case of lack of sufficient nursing care. Suction setup should be ready and anesthetist should be informed prior to this step
- Depending on the indication, appropriate sized tracheostomy tube should be inserted. For acute airway obstruction, a metal tube is sufficient and in case of need for ventilation a cuffed tube can be inserted
- Fixing of the tubes can be done by tying reef knots from the tube around the neck. The knots must be sufficiently tight enough to prevent accidental dislocation of the tubes. The knots must be tied with neck flexed
- The lateral ends of the incised wound can be sutured and sufficient space around the tube will minimize subcutaneous emphysema.
- In emergency, a vertical skin incision from the level of cricothyroid membrane to the suprasternal notch done, finger dissection can be pushed inferiorly to expose the upper three tracheal rings. A midline vertical incision can be done over trachea (2nd and 3rd tracheal rings) and with the help of tracheal dilator or hemostat, the tracheostomy tube can be inserted.[7]

POSTOPERATIVE CARE

Positioning

Initially, patient is placed in a high Fowler's position to minimize edema, to maximize the ease of coughing and deep breathing, to facilitate suctioning and to minimize discomfort (Figure 4.6). For infants, they can be placed in an infant seat in a semi-upright position and head must be supported in a neutral position immediately postoperatively.

Monitoring

Blood pressure, pulse rate and respiratory rate should be recorded every 15 minutes until patient becomes stable and every one hour, for the first 24 hours. Indications of respiratory distress during postoperative period are:

- Restlessness
- Change in blood pressure
- Increased respiratory rate

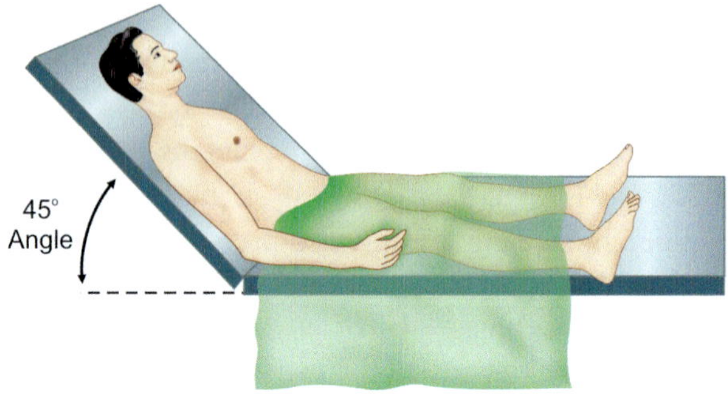

Figure 4.6 High-Fowler's position

- Increased pulse rate
- Retraction of intercostal spaces
- Use of accessory muscles
- Prolonged respiration
- Nasal flaring and head bobbing in infants.

The appearance of these signs should motivate tube patency assessment.

Suctioning

The patient's vital signs and breath sounds should be monitored before the attempt of suctioning. The lowest amount of negative pressure needed to remove secretions should be used to avoid trauma to the tracheal mucosa. Appropriate sized suction catheter should be used in relation to age of the patient and size of the tracheostomy tube used. The diameter of catheter should be half the internal diameter of the tracheostomy tube. In intubated patients, with more thick, tenacious and secretions, 2–3 mL of normal saline can be instilled into the tracheostomy tube before suctioning.

Aseptic measures are used in suction, changing of the tubes and dressing of the wound. Inner tube is changed as often as necessary. Outer tube is not changed for minimum of 72 hours, since the tract is not formed yet. Few days later, the metal tube can be changed with a suitable portex tube.

When patients need assisted ventilation, suitable cuffed tracheostomy tube is to be used.

Low pressure, high volume cuffs will prevent tracheal stenosis at the cuff sight. Minimal leak technique is used for inflating the cuff. The cuff pressure should be less than about 25 mm of Hg—less than the tracheal capillary pressure so that the capillaries are not occluded, which leads to ischemic necrosis of the trachea which in turn may lead to tracheal stenosis.

The cuff should be deflated for 10 minutes every hour. Suction should be applied after deflation, since secretions from above the cuff may trickle down to the trachea.

Proper humidification or instilling sodium bicarbonate or saline into the trachea will prevent crusting. Y-connection and suction are used. Negative pressure suction for more than few seconds is avoided. Patient is hyperventilated with 100% oxygen before suctioning. Science studies shows that the chances of tracheal stenosis are more in patients with gastroesophageal reflux, measures to control and treat reflux are taken to reduce chances of subglottic and laryngotracheal stenosis.

Nursing care after tracheostomy is important that includes nursing care to prevent infection. Care has to be taken for eye, mouth and back. Feeding is done by nasogastric tube. Proper nourishment to the patient is kept up.[4]

Home Care for Tracheostomy

Requirements

- Appropriate-sized tracheostomy tubes and one a size smaller
- Neck ties
- Scissors (for cutting ties)
- Tube lubricant
- Sterile syringes and saline
- Dressing set
- Appropriate sized suction catheters and suction machine
- Heat and moisture exchangers/Swedish noses/nebulizers
- Speaking valves
- Gloves
- Stethoscope
- Saturation monitor
- Ambu-bag
- Portable oxygen cylinders.[2]

TYPES OF TRACHEOSTOMY TUBES

Choice of tracheostomy tubes can be done by assessing the following criteria:

- Diameter

  Age-appropriate-sized tracheostomy tube must be selected to alleviate various complications like frequent obstruction in the case of small-sized tube for age. Too large tracheostomy tubes may predispose to suprastomal collapse and increase the risk of granulations and stenosis
- Length

  Too lengthy tube will abut the carina and lead to mucosal injury and potentially subsequent scarring. Too short tube increases risk of accidental decannulation. Tube tip position should be assessed by chest X-ray, rigid bronchoscopy and flexible endoscope through lumen of the tube

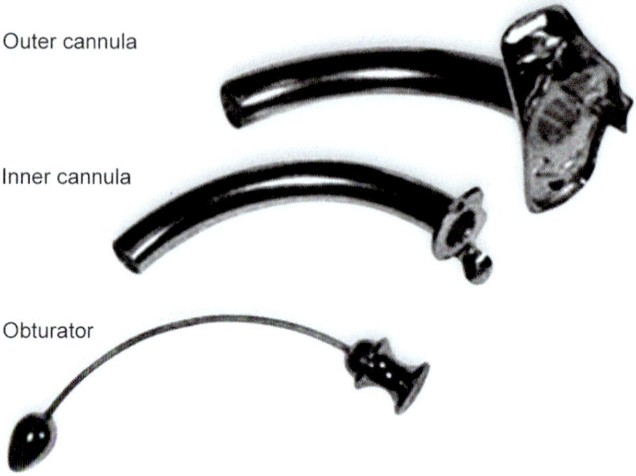

Figure 4.7 Metal tracheostomy tubes

- Material

  Silicone is most preferred due to relative flexibility compared to metal tubes. But in metal tubes (Figure 4.7), it is possible to achieve a smaller outside for the same internal diameter as a silicone tube
- Speaking valve

  Speaking valves are one-way valves, which allow inhalation through the tube but force air upwards through the glottis on exhalation, creating sufficient subglottic pressure to allow phonation. They also help in improving lung function and reduce aspiration. But small infants may have decreased tolerability towards the valves (Figure 4.8)
- Fenestration

  These tubes allow air to pass upwards to improve phonation. However, they may become a focus for granulation and mucosal trauma while suctioning
- Inner tube

  The advantage is that inner tube can be removed daily for cleaning and they can be available with integrated speaking valve. Disadvantage is that they reduce the tube diameter and are less practical in smaller children
- Cuff

  Two specific indications are when there is significant risk of aspiration or when there is decrease in lung compliance with intercurrent infection in a ventilated patient (Figure 4.9).[2]

There are more advanced models of tracheostomy tubes available viz, portex low pressure cuff tubes, NCC tubes with extra neck plate, RUSCH model tubes

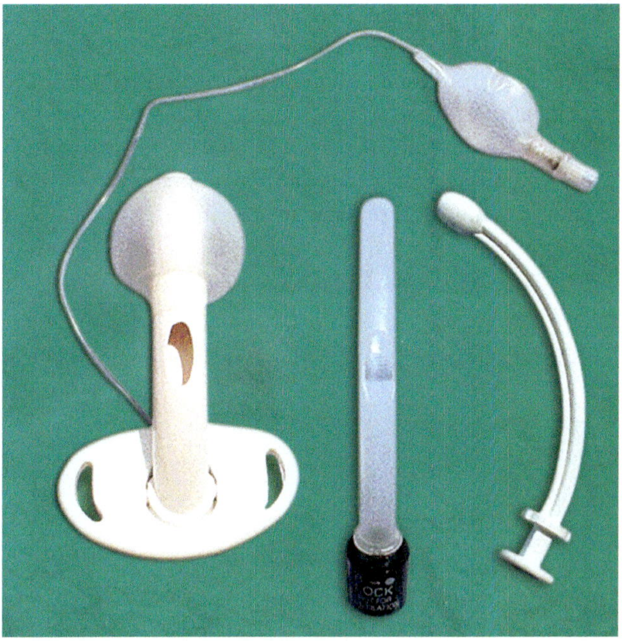

Figure 4.8 Nonmetallic portex tracheostomy tube with speaking valve

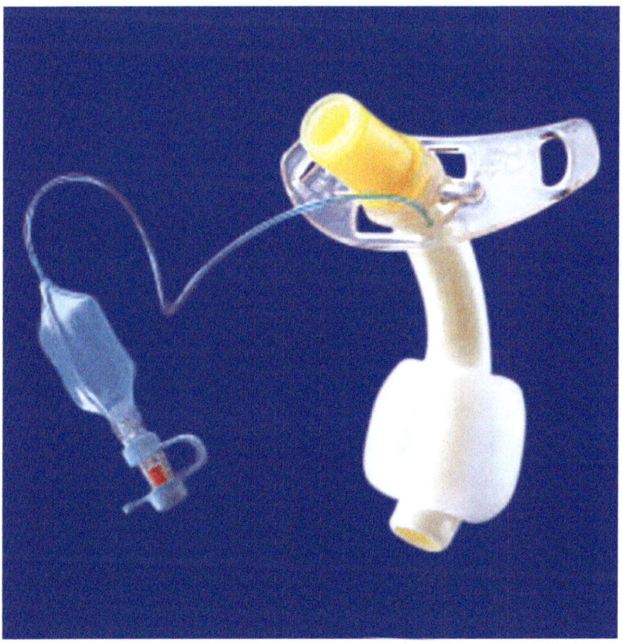

Figure 4.9 Nonmetallic portex tracheostomy tube (cuffed)

with super safety cuff, Molnlyeke-Steritex NL tube with flexible intratracheal portion—adjustable neck plate, built-in suction line, automatic cuff pressure regulating system, McGinn's tube with pressure limiting balloon, Lomholt design tubes with integrated suction, etc.[4]

A study made by Heather MS Coffman, Catherine J Rees with Shiley cuffed tubes and portex blue line ultrasuctionoid (BLUS), shows that the tubes with integrated subglottic suction port reduces incidence of aspiration and pneumonia.[8]

- Metallic tubes

  Koenig's tube, Durham's tube, Fuller's tube, Jackson's tube, etc.
- Nonmetallic tubes

  Portex tube, Bivona tube (Figure 4.10), Shiley tube (Figure 4.11), etc.

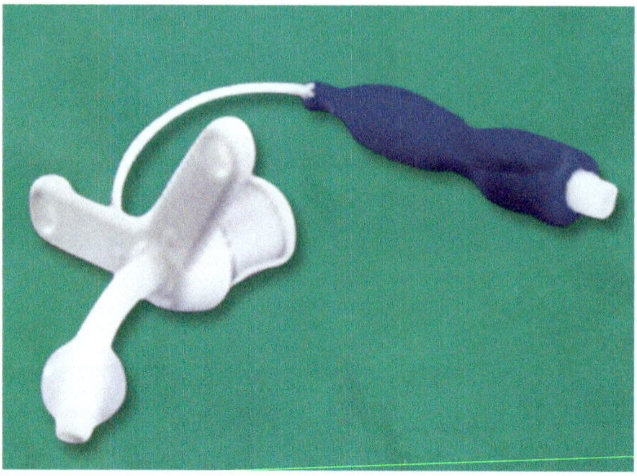

Figure 4.10 Bivona tracheostomy tube

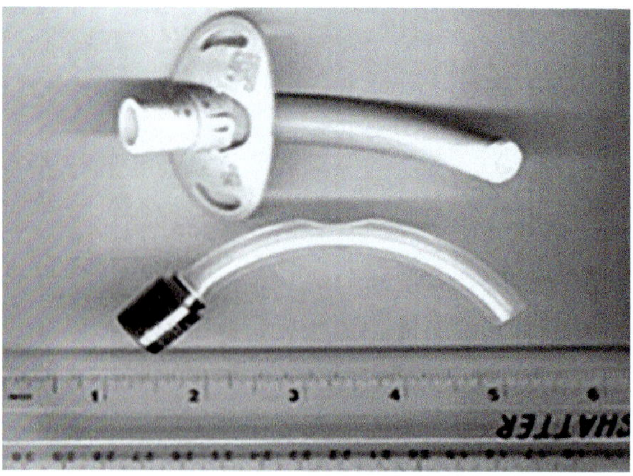

Figure 4.11 Shiley tracheostomy tube

COMPLICATIONS OF TRACHEOSTOMY

General

- Tube obstruction
- Accidental decannulation
- General surgical complications
- Death.

Immediate (During the Procedure)

- Hemorrhage from anterior jugular veins or thyroid gland
- Injury to recurrent laryngeal nerve
- Injury to pleura
- Injury to 1st tracheal ring or cricoid (leads to laryngotracheal stenosis).

Intermediate (Up to One Week of Surgery)

- Bleeding—postoperative, wound edge
- Surgical emphysema
- Pneumothorax
- Apnea
- Pneumomediastinum
- Collapse of the lung
- Respiratory tract infection
- Blocking of the inner tube
- Displacement of the outer tube
- Erosion of blood vessel—tracheoinnominate artery fistula.

Late (After One Week)

- Laryngeal stenosis
- Granulation
- Aphonia or speech delay
- Tracheitis sicca and crusting
- Pulmonary infection—atelectasis of lung
- Suprastomal collapse
- Bleeding
- Tracheal stenosis
- Decannulation problems
- Tracheomalacia.[2,6,7,9]

TRACHEOSTOMY IN THE PEDIATRIC PATIENTS

Incision can be simple vertical over the trachea without excising anterior tracheal wall or creating Bjork flap, preferably over the 3rd and 4th tracheal rings. Dissection in small children can be done with monopolar or bipolar cautery in small children. Mere dilation of vertical incision over trachea can be done with placing two sutures each on either side of the incision to serve as guide in case of misplacing of the tube. The suture can be removed in 3 or 4 days after tracheostomy.

PERCUTANEOUS TRACHEOSTOMY

This procedure began as mini tracheostomy for evaluation of bronchial secretions in the care of critically ill postoperative patients. It evolved as a procedure for bedside tracheostomy of critically ill patients who need long-term ventilation in the intensive care unit. It can be done as a blind procedure or with bronchoscopic guidance. Several kits are available for this procedure. Familiarity with specific kit and its use is crucial before actual application. The limitation being that it requires more time. It is a usual procedure for an already ventilated patient in the intensive care unit.

It may be a hazardous procedure in those patients with short, thick necks and goiters but those hazards can be overcomed by endoscopic control of the procedure.

There are various techniques available such as Ciaglia technique, Schachner (Rapitrach) technique, translaryngeal tracheostomy (Fantoni's technique), Percu twist method, Crigg's technique.

Contents of percutaneous tracheostomy kit (Figure 4.12)

- Scalpel
- 14 G intravenous needle and cannula

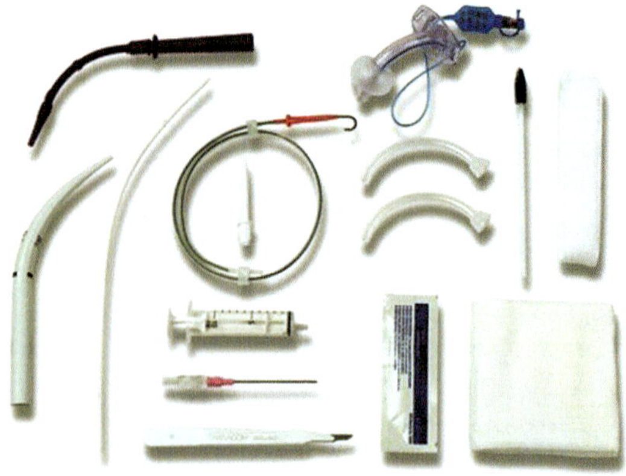

Figure 4.12 Percutaneous tracheostomy kit

- 10 mL syringe
- Flexible Teflon-coated guidewire
- Plastic dilator
- Pair of tracheal dilating forceps (with groove in the jaws to allow passage of guidewire)
- Tracheostomy tube with a hollow obturator to slide over the guidewire (cuffed).

Ciaglia Technique

- The procedure requires two trained personnel, one to perform the procedure and the other to maintain patient's airway and circulation and to provide anesthesia
- Position: Patient placed with neck extended with pillow or sand bag under the shoulders
- Complete monitoring of the patient with pulse oximetry, capnography, electrocardiography and blood pressure is essential
- Suprasternal notch and surface markings of the laryngeal framework structures are marked
- Infiltration done with 10 mL of 1% lignocaine with 1:200,000 adrenaline
- 14 G cannula, attached to a syringe containing normal saline, is inserted at the midpoint of distance between lower border of cricoid cartilage and suprasternal notch (Figure 4.13). Aspiration has to be done at regular intervals while advancing the cannula
- Successful tracheal puncture is indicated by sudden air entry in the syringe (Figure 4.14)
- Syringe removed and guidewire passed through the cannula.
- Dilator is then passed through guidewire into anterior wall of trachea to achieve adequate opening
- Tracheal dilator passed through guidewire to dilate the soft tissues and the tracheal wall (Figure 4.15)
- Finally obturator and tracheostomy tube passed through guidewire, guide wire and obturator being removed and tracheostomy tube fixed by inflating the cuff and tube position confirmed by assessing air entry into both lungs (Figures 4.16 to 18).

The evolution of newer techniques in percutaneous tracheostomy has significantly reduced complications. In a study made by H Birbicer and colleagues who compared the newer Percu twist method with multidilational Ciaglia technique, have shown to have reduced postoperative complications in Percu twist technique which is a single step technique.

In an another study done by Karen M Kost, who compared Crigg's and Ciaglia technique, have found Ciaglia technique to have more precise surgery, relatively short operative time and with less complications.[12]

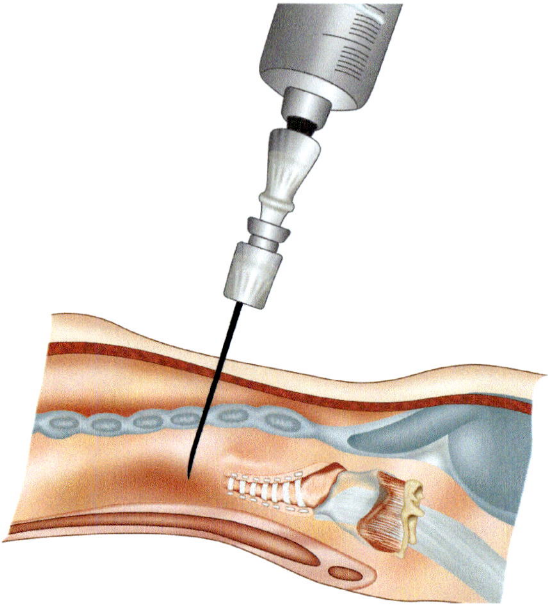

Figure 4.13 Percutaneous dilational tracheostomy (PDT technique) (Needle access of airway)

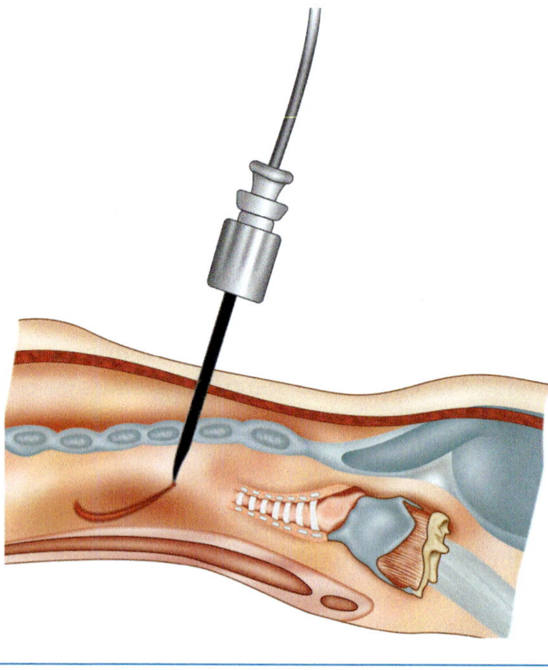

Figure 4.14 Percutaneous dilational tracheostomy (PDT technique) (Needle access of airway after blunt dissection of pretracheal tissues)

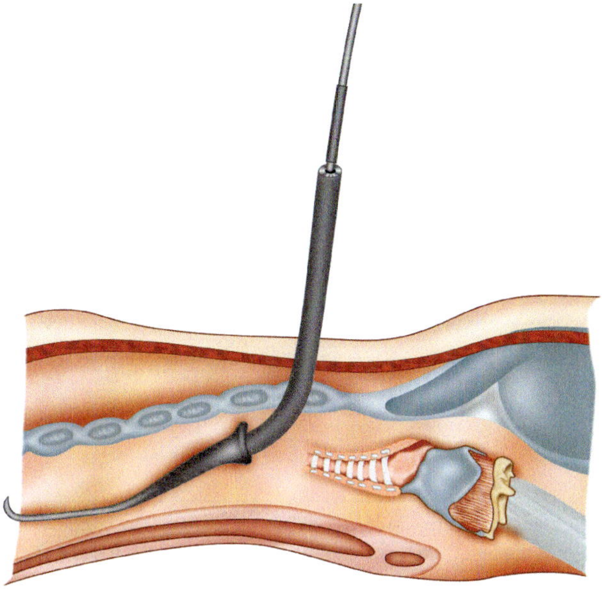

Figure 4.15 Percutaneous dilational tracheostomy (PDT technique) (Serial dilations are performed over the guidewire)

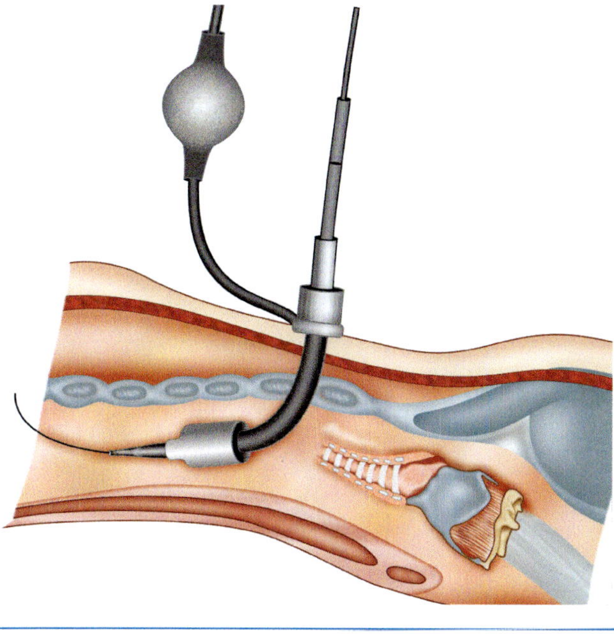

Figure 4.16 Percutaneous dilational tracheostomy (PDT technique) (A tracheostomy tube is inserted in the dilated passageway using a dilator as obturator over the guidewire)

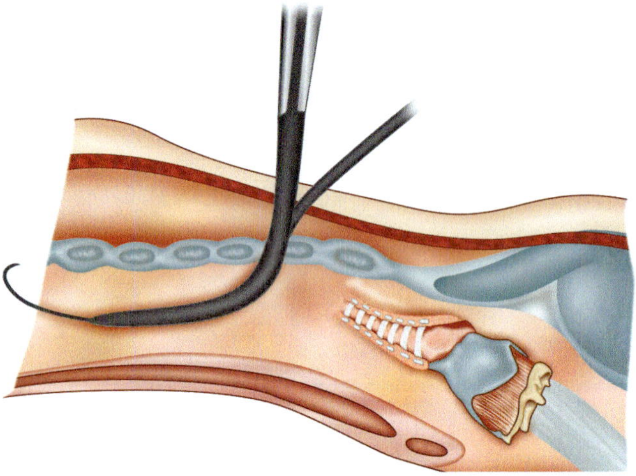

Figure 4.17 Guidewire dilating forceps (GWDF) technique (The guidewire dilator forceps are advanced along the Seldinger wire into the long axis of the trachea)

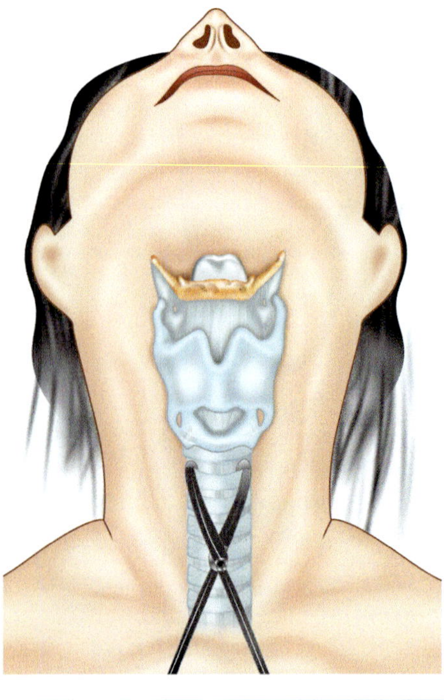

Figure 4.18 Guidewire dilating forceps (GWDF) technique (The guidewire dilator forceps enlarge the hole between tracheal rings)

Table 4.1 Percutaneous vs surgical tracheostomy

S. No.		Percutaneous tracheostomy	Surgical tracheostomy
1.	Procedure	Simple-dilational	Incised
2.	Bleeding	Less common	Relatively more common
3.	Duration	Lengthy	Relatively short
4.	Precision	Blind procedure	Relatively precise
5.	Personnel	Can be performed by non-otolaryngologists, emergency physicians, anesthetists, paramedical staff	Done by otolaryngologists

Contraindications

- Children less than 12 years of age
- Anatomic abnormality of trachea
- Pulsating palpable blood vessel over tracheostomy site
- Short or obese neck
- History of difficult intubation
- Limited ability to extend cervical spine
- Previous surgery over neck or larynx
- Acute infection over tracheostomy site
- Platelet count <40000/cubic mm
- Prothrombin time >1.5 times control
- Bleeding time >10 minutes
- Enlarged thyroid gland.[6,10]

According to T Veenith et al., percutaneous tracheostomy in ICU has less incidence of complications compared to conventional surgical technique (Table 4.1).[11]

CRICOTHYROIDOTOMY

Emergency cricothyroidotomy is time-honored, rapid method for securing the airway and has saved many lives. If the requirement for tracheostomy is needed, conversion to a standard tracheostomy within 24 to 48 hours is advisable.

Various steps involved in the procedure are:

- Extending the neck
- Palpating the cricoid arch and entering just above it
- Entering larynx just above the cricoid
- Midline incision done using either blade or intravenous cannula

- Blade can be rotated through 90 degree to keep the incision open
- Conversion to formal tracheostomy must be done as soon as possible.[10]

Contraindications

- Patients with increased risk of subglottic stenosis
- Pre-existing laryngeal disease
- Malignancy
- Inflammation near proximity
- Epiglottitis
- Abnormal anatomy of larynx
- Bleeding diathesis
- Infants and children.[6,10]

Complications

- Perichondritis
- Hypercapnea
- Subglottic edema
- Subglottic stenosis.

DECANNULATION

Decannulation may be considered when the original condition requiring tracheostomy has improved, however, to make decannulation successful, the patient should maintain an adequate airway without tracheostomy tube in place.

Removal of tracheostomy doubles dead space and triples airway resistance. Decannulation can be done as:

- Staged decannulation—Done in various stages like reducing the cuff pressure, changing to a smaller sized tube, etc.
- Immediate decannulation—Can be done as single step procedure preferably in a controlled setting. It should be avoided in cases where oral intubation is not possible (e.g. Treacher-Collins syndrome).

After decannulation, a fistula may persist between trachea and skin, which may discharge tracheal secretions called tracheocutaneous fistula. The fistula can be allowed for 6–12 months before formal closure, which is done with transfixion sutures.[2]

CONCLUSION

Otolaryngologist plays a vital role in the development of speech and language in tracheostomized patients. Referral to speech pathologist should be initiated after tracheostomy. It is the duty of the surgeon to alleviate various psychological and social problems in the patients and motivate family support in tracheostomized patients.

REFERENCES

1. Liess BD, Scheidt TD, Templer JW. The difficult airway. Otolaryngol Clin N Am. 2008;41:567-80.
2. Pracy P, Saunders M. Tracheostomy and home care. In: Scott-Brown's Otorhinolaryngology, Head and Neck Surgery, 7th edition. 1194-1209,2292-304.
3. Schneider GT, Christensen NP, Doerr TD. Early tracheostomy in the elderly results in less Pneumonia. Otolaryngol Head and Neck Surg. 2008;139:70-1.
4. Myers EN, Stool SE, Johnson JT. Tracheotom. The University of Michigan Churchill Livingstone. 2008.
5. Amygdalou A, Dimopoulos G, Moukas M. Immediate postoperative effects of tracheotomy on respiratory function during mechanical ventilation. Crit Care. 2004; 8:R243-7.
6. Goldenberg D, Bhatti N. Management of the impaired airway in the adult; In: Cumming's Otolaryngology, Head and Neck Surgery, 7th edition. 1194-1209,2292-304.
7. Wright D. Tracheostomy and laryngotomy; In: Rob and Smith's Operative Surgery: Nose and Throat, 5th edition. 269-76.
8. Coffman HMS, Rees CJ. Proximal suction tracheostomy tube reduces aspiration volume. Otolaryngol Head and Neck Surg. 2008;138,441-5.
9. Birbicer H, Doruk N. Percutaneous tracheostomy: A comparison of percu twist and multidilational techniques. Annals of Card Anaes. 2008;11(2).
10. Watkinson JC, Gaze MN, Wilson JA. Tracheostomy In: Stell and Maran's Head and Neck Surgery, 4th edition. 9,163-8.
11. Veenith T, Ganeshamoorthy S. Intensive care unit tracheostomy: a snapshot of UK practice. International Arch Med. 2008;1:21;10,1186/1755-7682-1-21.
12. Kost KM. Percutaneous tracheostomy: Comparison of Ciaglia and Criggs techniques; Crit Care. 2000;4:143-6.

CHAPTER

5 Vertigo

Any movement or sense of movement, either in the individual himself or in the external object that involves a defect, real or seeming in the equilibrium of the body.

Gower

Vertigo may be defined basically as a data mismatch in the sensory mechanism of the balance system consisting of visual, vestibular, acoustic, proprioceptive, CNS and peripheral nervous system.

Claussen

INTRODUCTION

Maintenance of balance is essential for the management of daily activities. This complex physical function depends on integrated, finely tuned processing of sensory inputs by the brain provided by the vestibular, visual and proprioceptive systems as well as by the cognitive system. Any disturbance in the integrative process of these systems will lead to "vertigo". The magnitude of prevalence and incidence of vertigo describes its importance. It is being reported to occur in 25% of middle-aged population and about 40% in elderly. In addition, by the age of 75 years, dizziness is the most common cause for seeking medical advice and also ninth most common cause for primary care physician visits. Improper diagnosis of vertigo at an emergency setup leads to unnecessary wasting of time and cost to patients. Vertigo not only represents a cardinal symptom for vestibular disorders, but also is furthermore associated with a wide spectrum of diseases. Vertigo may also appear in association with various organic diseases or may have a psychogenic origin. Vertigo imposes great limitations on patients' ability to meet their daily responsibilities, which results in a self-perceived decrease in quality of life. Vertiginous patients are also prone to frequent falls and thus injuries. Eventually, their insecurity about standing and loss of self-confidence may lead to immobilization. A sound knowledge on the pathophysiology and causes of vertigo is, therefore, very essential in diagnosing and treating the same.

FUNCTIONAL ANATOMY

Vestibular system is divided as peripheral and central. Central vestibular system consists of vestibular nuclei, connections of vestibular nuclei to cerebellum, spinal cord, extra ocular motor nuclei. Peripheral vestibular system consists of ear labyrinth.

The labyrinth consists of vestibule and semicircular canals and their projections into the brainstem (Figure 5.1). Utricle and saccule constitutes the vestibule. The labyrinth has two parts—bony and membranous. It is the membranous part which harbors hair cells that sense the motion of head. The impulses from superior and horizontal semicircular canals are carried by superior vestibular nerve and from posterior semicircular canal by the inferior vestibular nerve. The impulses are generated in the nerves by the inertia involving the hair cells in the various parts in labyrinth due to movement of endolymph. The utricle and saccule sense gravitational orientation and linear acceleration and semicircular canals detect change in the angular acceleration of the head. In simpler terms, semicircular canals act as velocity transducers during high velocity impulsive head movements to stabilize vision.

The sensory impulses, from the labyrinth, travel through the vestibular nerve to reach the Scarpa's ganglion similar to spiral ganglion, which receives auditory, impulses. From Scarpa's ganglion, the impulses are relayed to vestibular nuclei (Figure 5.2). There are 4 vestibular nuclei namely; superior, inferior, medial and lateral (Table 5.1).

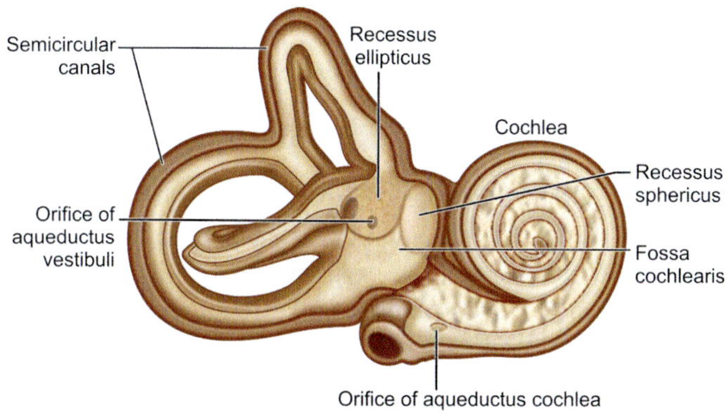

Figure 5.1 Anatomy of labyrinth

Table 5.1 Types of vestibular nuclei and their locations

Nuclei	*Location*
Superior (Bechterew nucleus)	Pons
Inferior (Spinal nucleus)	Lower medulla
Medial (Schwalbe nucleus, dorsal nucleus, chief vestibular nucleus)	Medulla (floor of fourth ventricle)
Lateral (nucleus of Deiters)	Upper medulla

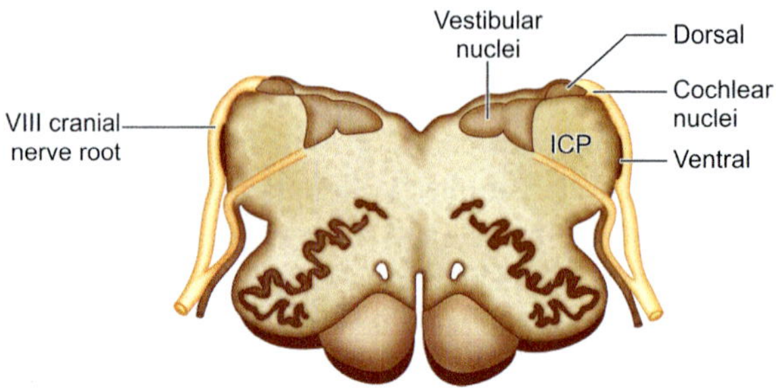

Figure 5.2 Location of vestibular nucleus

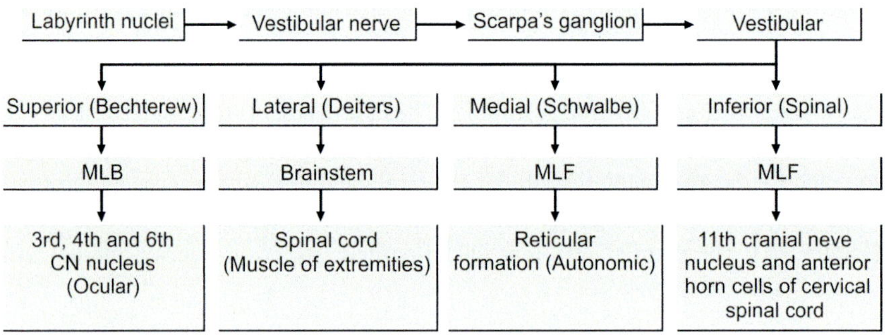

Figure 5.3 Functional anatomy of vestibular system (the complexity of balance). (MLB, medial longitudinal bundle; MLF, medial longitudinal fasciculus)

The superior vestibular nuclei relay impulses to medial longitudinal bundle (MLB) and hence, to the 3rd, 4th and 6th cranial nerve nuclei. Similarly, from the lateral vestibular nuclei impulses are transmitted to brainstem from where it reaches spinal cord to control muscles of extremities. Medial and inferior vestibular nuclei relay information to medial longitudinal fasciculus (MLF) and then to reticular formation and 11th cranial nerve nucleus, respectively (Figure 5.3).

ACUTE VERSUS CHRONIC VERTIGO

Acute vertigo is the common cause of frequent visit to emergency departments. Vertigo of acute onset usually results from pathology associated with vestibular nerve or the labyrinth. Acute attacks of vertigo are well-defined, isolated spells of vertigo with a distinct onset and offset, whereas chronic vertigo is defined as a continuous or chronic sensation. Recurrent attacks of vertigo are addressed as chronic vertigo.

ETIOLOGY

Vertigo presents with varied and diversified etiologies. There are about 69 different causes documented by Holt & Thomas in 1976. Oosterveld in 1997 reported that more than 100 different disorders are responsible for the occurrence of vertigo. Janet Wilson in 1997 have found that for about 88% of the cases, there can be more than one diagnosis and in about 71% of the cases, the cause can be a central vascular disease.

The causes of vertigo are categorized as follows:

- Organic
  - Peripheral causes
    - Meniere's disease
    - Labyrinthitis
    - BPPV—Benign paroxysmal positional vertigo
    - Ototoxicity
    - Perilymph fistula
    - Vestibular neuritis
    - Vestibular Schwannoma
    - Superior semicircular canal dehiscence syndrome
    - Trauma to the temporal bone
    - Cogan's syndrome
    - Otitic syphilis
    - Recurrent vestibulopathy
  - Central
    - Intracranial complications of otitis media
    - Transient ischemic attack (TIA) and stroke related disorders
    - Multiple sclerosis
    - Sarcoidosis
    - Basilar migraine
    - Friedreich's ataxia
    - Spinocerebellar ataxia
    - Craniocervical junction disorders (Arnold-Chiari malformations)
    - Diabetes mellitus
    - Hypothyroidism
    - Hypoventilation
    - Hypoglycemia
    - Alcohol intoxication
    - Parkinson's disease
    - Normal pressure hydrocephalus
    - Epilepsy

- Head trauma
- Epileptic vertigo
- Barré-Liéou syndrome
- Behcet's syndrome
- Post-meningitis/encephalitis
- Cerebrovascular disorder
  - Vertebrobasilar insufficiency
  - Subclavian steal syndrome
  - Wallenberg's syndrome (LMS)
  - Lateral pontine (Foville's) syndrome
  - Medial pontine (Millard Gubler) syndrome

- Functional

  Psychogenic origin—Panic syndromes, agoraphobia.

  Among these causes, except vestibular Schwannoma and ototoxicity, all are cause of acute vertigo.

PATHOPHYSIOLOGY

In a normal labyrinth, rapid eye movement to one side will cause ipsilateral increase in the input from the labyrinth and at the same time the input from contralateral labyrinth decreases (Figure 5.4). These inputs are interpreted by the brainstem that process the inputs and brings occulomotor effect resulting in deviation of eyeballs as equal and opposite to head movement.

However, at the same time, in case of severe unilateral vestibular loss, there will be only a contralateral input and the brainstem will interpret the input as circular motion in the direction of remaining side (Figure 5.5). Therefore, the effect will be driving of eyeballs slowly to the impaired side and quick snap back to the intact side. So, spontaneous nystagmus will be directed opposite to the lesion in case of peripheral vestibular failure. In case of bilateral vestibular loss, there will be bilateral loss of semicircular canal inputs and so no asymmetry is sensed by brainstem, which results in deficient vestibulo-ocular reflex (VOR) (Figure 5.6). This deficiency leads to blurring of vision because of slippage of images across the retina.

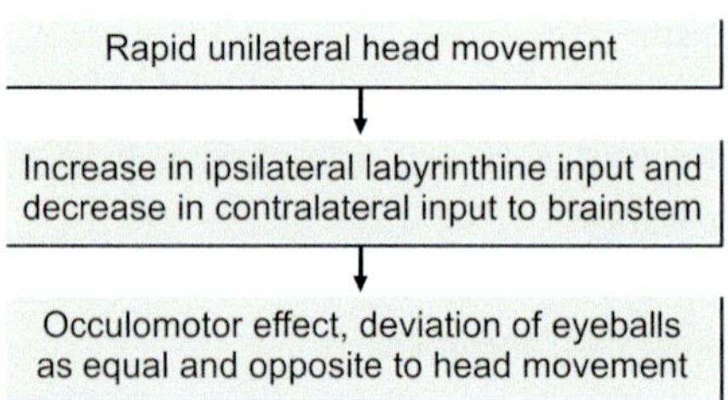

Figure 5.4 Normal labyrinth

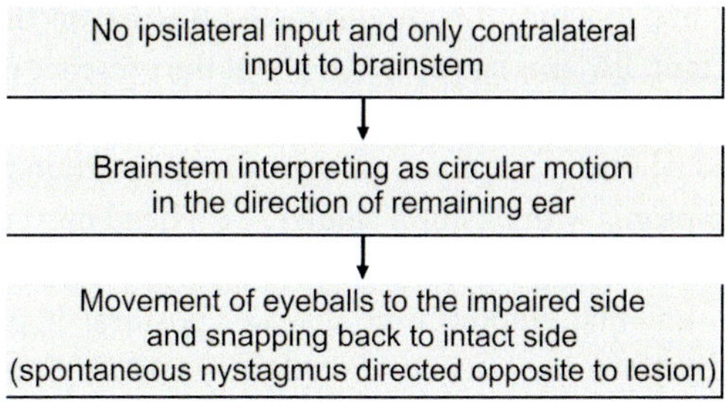

Figure 5.5 Unilateral severe vestibular loss

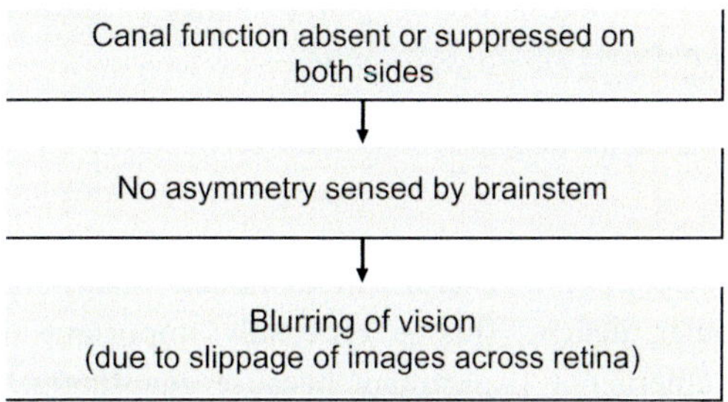

Figure 5.6 Bilateral severe vestibular loss (bilateral loss of semicircular canal inputs)

PRESENTATION

The various presentations of vertigo are as follows:

- Dizziness
- Rocking sensation
- Rotating sensation
- Instability
- Nausea and vomiting
- Tendency to fall
- Black out
- Collapse
- Lifting sensation
- Floating
- Tilting
- Light headedness
- Visual disorientation.

HISTORY AND EXAMINATION

History indicates to provisional diagnosis in 80% of cases. The two symptoms that correlate well with vestibular disorder are vertigo and oscillopsia (perception that stationary objects are moving). Eliciting detailed history on the presentation of dizziness is important. Patients can be asked about the presence of illusory sense of motion, if present whether internal or there is movement in the environment, they should be enquired whether symptoms are episodic or continuous, precipitation or aggravation of symptoms with postural change, with head movement or following pressure or sound stimuli, underlying medical problems like thyroid disorders, diabetes mellitus, anemia, autoimmune disease, postural hypotension, cardiac arrhythmias, medications use, anxiety disorders, panic syndromes, agoraphobia (fear for open, large, crowded environment). Emphasis should be made about eliciting associated symptoms with dizziness like, aural fullness, tinnitus, dysarthria, diplopia, sweating, dyspnea and palpitations. Hallmark of peripheral vestibular disease is distinct nature of spell, presence of auditory symptoms and absence of central nervous system symptoms.

The most important in the diagnosis of vertigo is an unhurried and detailed history.

AG Kerr

With careful bedside clinical examination, one can usually diagnose a unilateral peripheral vestibular deficit. This is especially important in those patients evaluated in the emergency department because quantitative caloric testing is rarely immediately available. The mandatory examinations to be performed are:

- Cranial nerve assessment
- Spontaneous nystagmus
- Gaze-evoked nystagmus
- Positional nystagmus
- Hallpike induced nystagmus
- Post head-shake nystagmus
- Head thrust test
- Dynamic visual acuity test
- Cerebellar limb tests
- Gait observation
- Examination of pursuit and saccadic eye movements.

Nystagmus can be elicited on clinical examination, which can be spontaneous or evoked. Spontaneous nystagmus is seen when there is a static imbalance in tonic levels of neural activity in pathways arising from semicircular canals. Head-shake nystagmus should be examine if there is absence of spontaneous nystagmus. Head-shake maneuver can be performed by asking the patient to shake-head side to side 20–30 cycles and stop abruptly. It can be also done using vertical head movement. Examination should be done to detect Skew deviation by alternate cover test, which is finding vertical corrective movement of the eyeballs while moving a card covered to one eye to the other. Other findings like head-shaking nystagmus, head-thrust nystagmus should also be documented.

Caloric tests are of essential value till today in diagnosing peripheral vestibular disorders and helps in differentiating peripheral from central vestibular disorders. It can be done by making the patient lie on a bed with head elevated to 30 degree from the horizontal level and infiltrating the ear canal with cold and hot water or saline and simultaneous interpretation of nystagmus in the eyeballs. Normally, the cold water causes eyeball movement to the opposite side and warm water towards the same side. The limitations of caloric tests are, it tests the function of horizontal semicircular canal and the function of the other canals can be over looked. Moreover, caloric test stimuli are not physiological and are less tolerated by patients.

Positional tests like Dix-Hallpike maneuver (Figure 5.7), helps in measuring canal paresis and directional preponderance. For estimating canal paresis, the formula of Jongkees et al. can be used: {[(R 30°C + R 44°C)–(L 30°C + L 44°C)]/[(R 30°C + R 44°C + L 30°C + L 44°C)]} × 100 where, for example, R 30°C is the maximum slow phase velocity of nystagmus induced by the caloric irrigation of the right ear canal with 30°C warm water. Vestibular paresis was defined as >25% asymmetry between the right- and left-side responses.

Dynamic visual acuity, Valsalva-induced nystagmus, hyperventilation-induced nystagmus, fistula test guides to diagnosis of bilateral vestibulopathy, craniocervical abnormalities, demyelinating disorders of vestibular nerve, labyrinthine fistula, respectively. Vestibulospinal examination tests like Romberg's test, tandem walking, past pointing, stepping tests helps to exclude vestibulospinal imbalance in the diagnosis. Stepping tests are done by asking the patient to march in place with eyes closed and arms extended to the front.

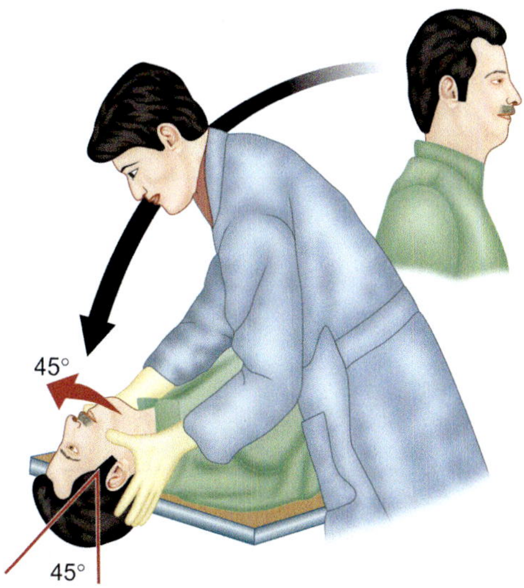

Figure 5.7 Dix-Hallpike test

Rotation Tests

Stimulating vestibular system by rotating the subject in a horizontal plane and observing the eye movement response that occurs as a result of stimulation of VOR. The response is proportional to the stimulus.

Other tests like smooth pursuit, which involves patient to track a sinusoidally moving target, optokinetic nystagmus and saccades are to be tested. Saccades are fast compensatory movement of the eyeballs. Additionally, head impulse test, head heave tests are found to precipitate nystagmus in patients with unilateral vestibular loss, mainly in those people where spontaneous nystagmus was not elicitable. The head-impulse test was performed by rapidly rotating the patient's head (abrupt, high-acceleration rotations of about 20° amplitude) to the right and to the left. The head-heave test was performed by heaving the head of the

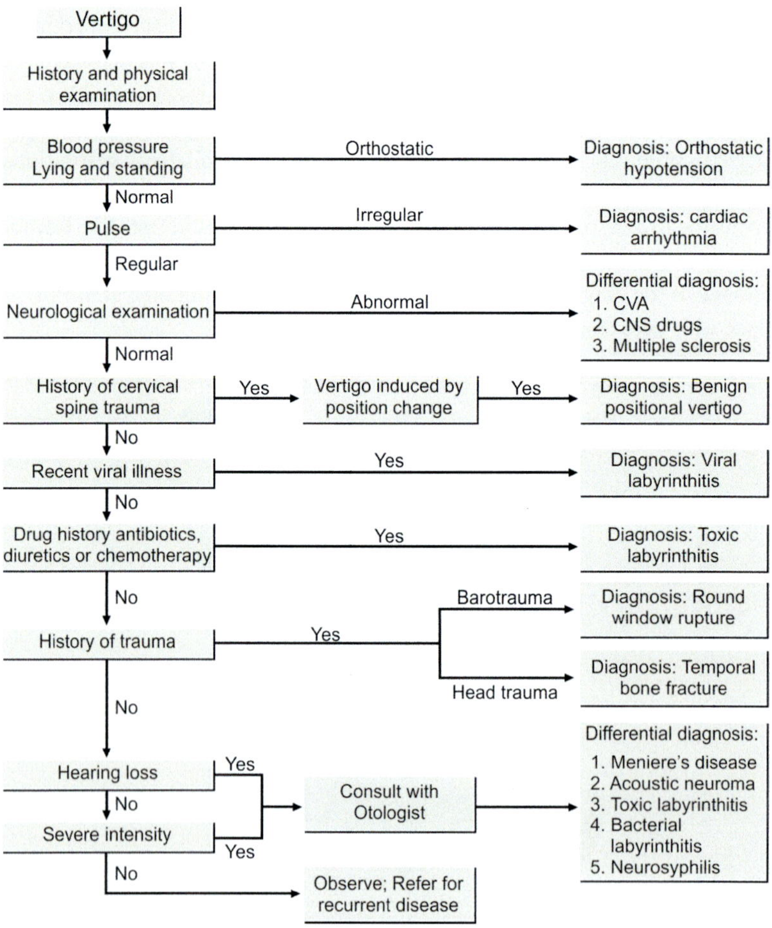

Figure 5.8 Algorithm of vertigo diagnosis

patient rapidly (abrupt, high-acceleration interaural translations [heaves] of about 5–10 cm in excursion).

Marco Mandalà et al. have documented in their study of 68 patients with unilateral vestibular neuritis that head impulse test has diagnostic value and also the patients with head impulse have relatively low prognosis.

CENTRAL VERSUS PERIPHERAL VERTIGO (TABLE 5.2)

Table 5.2 Comparison between peripheral and central vertigo

Sl. No.	*Features*	*Peripheral*	*Central*
1.	Occurrence	Episodic	May be constant
2.	Severity	Proportionate to nystagmus	Disproportionate
3.	Nystagmus axis	Horizontal	Rotationary or variable
4.	Type of nystagmus	Slow and Ist phase	Irregular and equal phase
5.	Nystagmus latency	10 to 20 seconds	None
6.	Nystagmus direction	Single	Changing
7.	Nystagmus duration	Brief	Long
8.	Nystagmus fatigability	Yes	No
9.	Nystagmus habituation	Yes	No
10.	Associated aural symptoms	Yes	Possible
11.	Neurological sysmptoms/ signs	Absent	Possible

DIAGNOSIS

Most vertigo patients can be diagnosed by precise documentation of duration of symptoms and presentation of each episode.

- Vertigo lasting for seconds—most probably BPPV from downmost ear
- Vertigo lasting for minutes—endolymphatic hydrops, TIA, migraine, perilymph fistula
- Vertigo lasting for hours—vestibular neuritis, migraine, stroke
- Variable presentation—inner ear fistulae, barotrauma, superior semicircular dehiscence syndrome.

Vestibulopathies most often causes fluctuating or episodic symptoms and similarly vertigo occurring due to psychogenic syndromes will mimic vestibulopathies. BPPV is the most common cause of vertigo of peripheral origin. Patients present often with history of positional vertigo, i.e. vertigo presents mainly on rolling over in bed, tilting the head backward and towards the ear. Aural fullness, tinnitus with vertigo may guide the diagnosis to Meniere's disease. Dysarthria, diplopia and paresthesias, if associated with vertigo, should be suspected with vertebrobasilar insufficiency. Sweating, dyspnea, palpitations often accompany psychogenic panic attacks. If dizziness is associated with hearing loss and/or tinnitus, cochlear or 8th cranial nerve pathology should be suspected. If there are associated brainstem, cerebellar and basal ganglia symptoms, neurological disease must be suspected. Anxiety, GI symptoms, palpitations, breathlessness and angina are associated with dizziness, the possibility of anemia, CVS disorders, thyroid disorders, diabetes mellitus should be thought.

88% of cases have more than one diagnosis.

Prof Janet Wilson

On examination, transient, torsional nystagmus point towards the diagnosis of BPPV and horizontal, contralateral, torsional nystagmus direct the diagnosis to Meniere's disease. During horizontal head shaking, rotatory nystagmus indicates the presence of unilateral labyrinthine dysfunction and presence of vertical nystagmus during horizontal head shaking implies the presence of central lesion. Caloric testing helps in diagnosing various peripheral vestibular disorders.

- Decreased caloric response on affected side—unilateral vestibular dysfunction
- Hyperactive caloric response—early Meniere's disease, central vestibular lesion.

In Dix-Hallpike test, presence of canal paresis indicates that the lesion is mostly in peripheral vestibular organs. Directional preponderance may be due to peripheral or central. Impaired VOR and impaired OKN are mainly due to central cause. Spontaneous nystagmus can be due to peripheral or central cause. Positional nystagmus of less than 30 seconds duration will be probably due to peripheral cause. Positional nystagmus fatigues in peripheral vestibular lesions.

Similarly, during vestibulospinal examination, tendency to fall to the affected side may represent Meniere's disease. Stepping tests are very useful in detecting early Meniere's disease. Abnormality of saccades implies CNS pathology (provided intact function of extraocular muscles). Overshooting saccade may be due to cerebellar disease and undershooting saccade indicates brainstem or basal ganglia lesions. Impaired pursuit may, sometimes due to CNS pathology.

INVESTIGATIONS

In spite of the most sophisticated diagnostic tests, there is often much uncertainty in making a diagnosis of vertigo and also not one single test leads to a definite conclusion as the vestibular system evades examination with persistent arrogance.

Electro-oculography (EOG), Electronystagmography (ENG) and Videonystagmography

ENG records eye movements objectively during examination and EOG is based on corneoretinal potential, i.e. it measures the electric signal arising from the inner ear in response to auditory stimulation. In Meniere's disease, EOG shows high SP:AP ratio, i.e. >0.35. (SP—summation potential, AP—action potential).

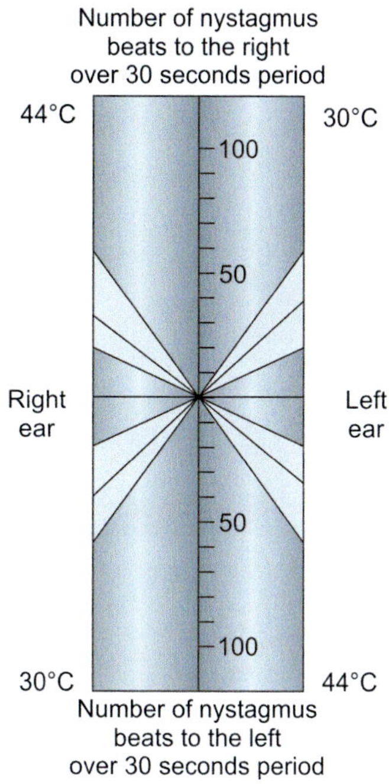

Figure 5.9 Butterfly chart

In a study done by G. Guidetti et al., in comparing normal clinical examination, with Frenzel glasses and videonystagmography for assessing the nature of nystagmus in OPD setting, they have concluded with the findings that videonystagmography is the method of choice.

A butterfly chart can be drawn based on culmination frequency of caloric test and spontaneous nystagmus by electronystagmography (Figure 5.9). The chart is divided into 4 quadrants. The values of culmination frequency for the 4 caloric tests (right hot, right cold, left hot and left cold) are plotted in the chart. Each quadrant in the chart is divided into 3 zones. Middle zone representing normalcy and hyperactive if the culmination frequency is above 59 beats/30 seconds and hypoactive if it is below 22 beats/30 seconds. The chart can also be used to plot spontaneous nystagmus.

- Auditory brainstem response testing
- Craniocarpography
- Optokinetic nystagmus test:

This test involves the subject to focus moving objects and simultaneously recording eye movements objectively

- Babinski-Weil test
- Computerized dynamic posturography (CDP) (Figure 5.10):

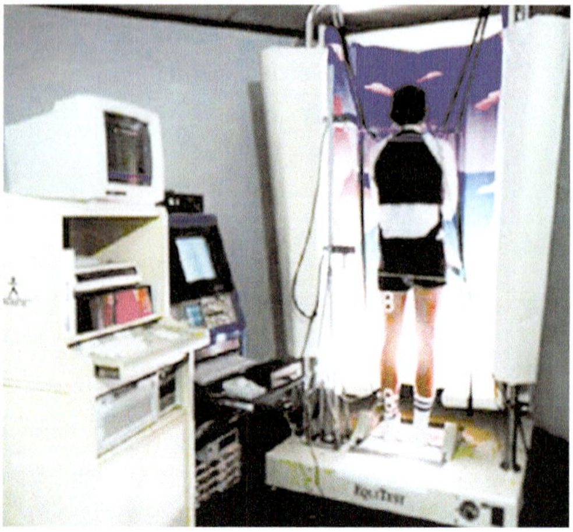

Figure 5.10 Dynamic posturography

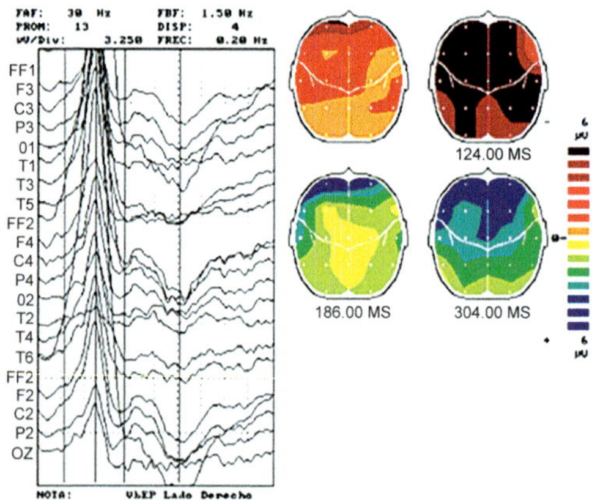

Figure 5.11 Vestibular evoked myogenic potential test

This test attempts to stress the ability to preserve equilibrium by removing or altering the information normally available from the visual and proprioceptive systems

- Vestibular evoked myogenic potential test (VEMP) (Figure 5.11)
- Fukuda's test
- Brain electrical activity mapping (BEAM)
- Magnetic resonance imaging with gadolinium enhancement
- Positron emission tomography (PET) and single photon emission computed tomography (SPECT) scan
- Functional magnetic resonance imaging and BEAM with VEP.

No single vestibular function test pinpoint the exact diagnosis.

Prof WJ Oosterveld

VESTIBULAR INDEX

It is essential for evaluating severity of vestibular disease and also prognosis of the same. It is done by assessing the following:

- Vertigo at rest
- Postural vertigo
- Spontaneous/gaze nystagmus
- Vestibulospinal reflexes
- Positional tests
- Caloric tests.

The index is the sum of five possible degrees of intensity between 0 (no vertiginous complaints and normal findings on vestibular function tests) to 4 (severe vertiginous complaints and very gross abnormality on vestibular function tests) on the above six parameters.

TREATMENT (FIGURE 5.12)

Principles

- Treat the cause
- Suppress the vestibular system
- Suppress the emotional reaction
- Encourage compensation
- Surgery, if necessary
- Accept the problem
- Not any therapy gives a full protection against vertigo
- Not any drug act in all persons, at anytime, in any condition
- The treatment is nonsurgical in vast majority of cases.

The vast majority of the patient can be managed by drug therapy, physical therapy or adoption exercise and only few may need surgery.

Millind V Kirtane

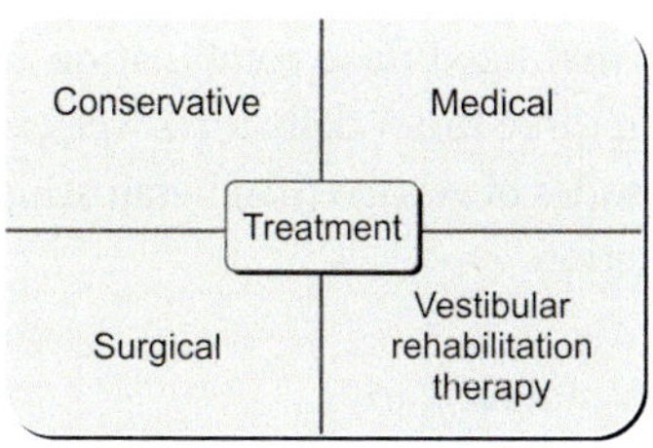

Figure 5.12 Treatment plan for vertigo

Conservative

Positional exercises provide remission in most cases of BPPV. Patients are advised to perform the exercises in the morning as their first task of the day. Patient is asked to sit upright at the edge of the couch and asked immediately to assume a lateral position, so as to provoke episode of vertigo. The patient is asked to retain the same position until the episode subsides and then asked to return to upright position. Patient is asked to perform this maneuver 2–3 times a day, up to the period where no response to exercise occurs. For Meniere's disease, dietary restriction in sodium is very essential. Bed rest with head elevation and avoidance of physical strain such as blowing of nose, etc., will arrest symptoms in perilymph fistula. Prevention is the best management option available in case of vertigo due to ototoxicity.

Medical

Following are the list of agents that help to reduce the symptoms:

- Vasodilators: Betahistine, niacin, papaverine
- Vestibular suppressants: Cinnarizine, cyclizine, meclizine, buclizine, promethazine, dimenhydrinate, ginkgo biloba, diazepam, clonazepam
- Psychotropic drugs: Nortriptyline, lorazepam
- Viscosity reducing agents: Pentoxiphylline
- Anti-inflammatory agents: Corticosteroids, NSAIDs
- Diuretics: Hydrochlorothiazides, triamterene, acetazolamide
- Drugs for migraine: Sumatriptan, propranolol, gabapentin
- Anticholinergics: Glycopyrrolate, propantheline, atropine, scopolamine
- Ototoxic drugs: Streptomycin, gentamicin.

Treatment of Acute Vertigo

Oral: (duration—4 weeks)

- Diazepam: 2–5 mg thrice; daily
- Meclizine: 25 mg thrice; daily
- Promethazine: 25–50 mg thrice; daily
- Tapered steroid regimen—80 mg OD of prednisolone for 7 days and tapered dose for another 7 days (for early vestibular neuritis or consecutive Meniere's disease). It has been proved by Zdenek Cirek et al. in their study of 61 patients with otogenic vertigo that fixed dose combination of cinnarizine 20 mg and dimenhydrinate 40 mg three times daily for 4 weeks, provided more outcome in minimizing the episodes of vertigo than betahistine 12 mg given three times daily for the same duration.

Parenteral:

- Diazepam: 5–10 mg intramuscularly
- Droperidol: 2.5 mg intramuscularly
- Prochlorperazine: 25 mg per rectum

Parenteral route preferred in case of severe symptoms, unresponsive to oral medication. Careful respiratory monitoring should be done in case of parenteral route selection as these medications might depress respiratory system. Additionally for Meniere's disease, potassium sparing diuretic therapy with betahistine and intratympanic low dose gentamicin therapy can be tried. For vertigo due to psychogenic causes like anxiety, lorazepam 2 mg—thrice daily can be given.

Surgical

Only <5% of the patients will require surgery. Surgery is indicated in cases of acute vertigo from unilateral disease not responding to medical therapy.

Types

- Hearing preserving
- With hearing destruction.

Indications

- Meniere's disease (transmastoid labyrinthectomy, endolymphatic decompression)
- Perilymph fistula
- Labyrinthine fistula
- BPPV (singular neurectomy).

Surgery is indicated only when there is an irreversible disturbance of labyrinthine function.

Prof Alan G Kerr

Vestibular Rehabilitation Therapy (VRT)

Candidacy

- Stable lesions of peripheral or central vestibular system
- Poor central integration
- Abnormal motor function.

Exercises

- Cawthorne—cooksey exercises
- Brandt—daroff habituation exercises (Figure 5.13)
- Epley's reposition technique
- Semont's liberatory maneuver.

Epley's maneuver involves repositioning of free floating endolymph particles into posterior semicircular canals. Semont's maneuver is a type of office maneuver which can be performed by asking the patient to lie on affected side with head

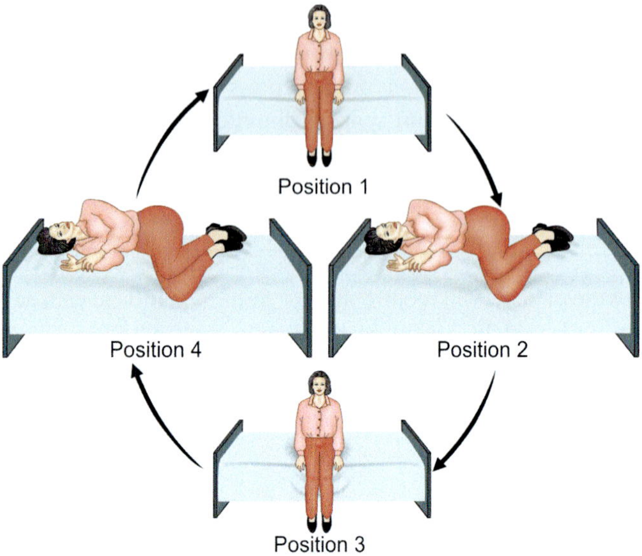

Figure 5.13 Brandt-Daroff exercise

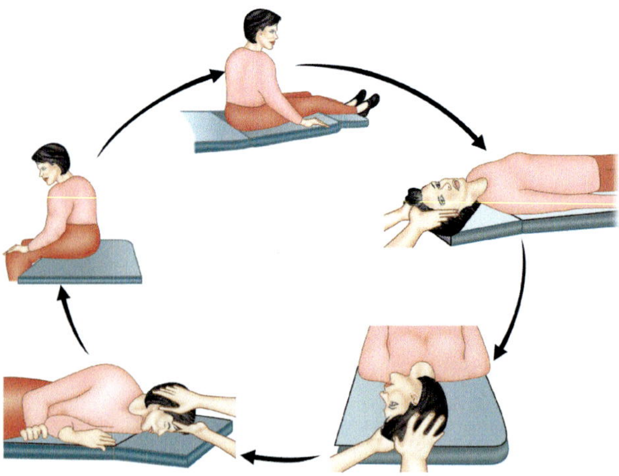

Figure 5.14 Epley's and Semont's maneuvers

propped 45 degree up and suddenly bringing back to upright posture with head turned 45 degree down (Figure 5.14).

Emmanuel Levrat and his colleagues, with their study of 278 patients diagnosed to have BPPV, have found the benefit of Semont's liberatory maneuver. They could demonstrate a 90.3% cure rate for BPPV.

The VRT can be used adjunctively after vestibular surgery, following head trauma and in psychogenic vertigo. It can be applied as a trial when there is uncertainty in diagnosis or in case of failure to improve unstable or progressive lesion. Patients with Meniere's disease are generally poor candidates for VRT.

QUALITY OF LIFE

Factors that affect quality of life in patients with vertigo are:

- Drug side effects
- Anxiety neurosis
- Agoraphobia
- Social impairment
- Depression
- "3 F" syndrome (Fear of Frequent Falling).

CONCLUSION

As per "American Institute of Health Statistics" data, 50% of all accident death from fall above 65 years are due to balance disorder. So "Essential geriatric care" is incomplete without proper strategy, protocol and facilities for diagnosis and management of vertigo. The need to develop a systematic, efficient and formal assessment strategy for the diagnosis of the symptom complex of dizziness or vertigo and disequilibrium is paramount in order to provide appropriate management and rehabilitation. The social consequences of vertigo and the increasing age of the population underline the importance of developing efficient antivertiginous therapies for both individual care and pharmacoeconomic reasons.

BIBLIOGRAPHY

1. Biswas A. Neurotology. 2ed edn. 2006:46-84.
2. Blatt PJ, Georgakakis GA, Herdman SJ, Clendaniel RA, Tusa RJ. The effect of the canalith repositioning maneuver on resolving postural instability in patients with benign paroxysmal positional vertigo. Am J Otol. 2000;21:356–63.
3. Bojrab DI, et al. Peripheral vestibular disorders. Jackler and Brackmann Neurootology. 36;629-650.
4. burman D, et al. A study on peripheral vertigo in a kolkata based hospital. Indian journal of otolaryngology and head and neck surgery. 2002 April-June;4.
5. Cirek Z, Schwarz M, Baumann W, Novotny M. Efficacy and tolerability of a fixed combination of cinnarizine and dimenhydrinate versus betahistine in the treatment of otogenic vertigo: A Double-Blind, Randomised Clinical Study. Clin Drug Invest. 2005;25(6):377-89.
6. Guidetti G, Monzani d, et al. Clinical examination of labyrinthine-defective patients out of the vertigo attack: sensitivity and specificity of three low-cost methods. Acta Otorhinolaryngol Ital. 2006;26:96-101.
7. Guilemany JM, et al. Clinical and epidemiological study of vertigo at an outpatient clinic. Acta Otolaryngol. 2004 Jan;124(1):49-52.
8. Halmagyi GM, et al. Vertigo: clinical syndromes. Scott-Browns otolaryngol Head Neck Surg. 7th ed. 3:240c;3748-90.
9. Harker, et al. Vestibular System. Cumming's Otolaryngol Head and Neck Surg. 4th edition. 4;3138-3320.

10. Hullar TE, Minor LB. et al. Vestibular physiology and Disorders of the Labyrinth. In: Glasscock-Shambaugh Surgery of the Ear, 5th edn. 2003;4:83-103.
11. Kerr AG. A symptomatic approach to vertigo. The Journal of Laryngology & Otology. 1983;97:813-5.
12. Levrat E, Melle G van, Monnier P, Maire R. Efficacy of the Semont Maneuver in Benign Paroxysmal Positional Vertigo. Arch Otolaryngol Head Neck Surg. 2003;129:629-33.
13. Mandalà M, et al. Effectiveness of careful bedside examination in assessment, diagnosis, and prognosis of vestibular neuritis. Arch Otolaryngol Head Neck Surg. 2008;134(2): 164-9.
14. Merchant SN, et al. Temporal bone studies of the human peripheral vestibular system. Normative vestibular hair cell data. Ann Otol Rhinol Laryngol Suppl. 2000 May;181:3-13.
15. Moulin T, Sablot D, Vidry E, Belahsen F, Berger E, lemounaud P, et al. Impact of emergency room neurologists on patient management and outcome. Eur Neurol. 2003;50:207-14.
16. Omahoney CF, Davies RA. Vestibular Investigations. Ludman and Wright Diseases of the Ear. 6th ed. 5;87-104.
17. Shepard NT, Solomon D. Practical issues in the management of dizzy and balance disorder patient. Otolaryngol Clin North Am. 2000;33(3):455-672.
18. Wilson JA, Colledge NR. The prevalence and characteristics of dizziness in an elderly community. Age Ageing. 1994 Mar;23(2):117-20.

CHAPTER

6 Diagnosis and Treatment of Headache and Facial Pain

INTRODUCTION

Aristotle had described pain as the passion of soul and Sherrington has described pain as a psychological adjunct to an imperative protective reflex. Whereas pain is the most common symptom in the body, headache is the commonest of all conditions. As per the International Headache Society (IHS), it has the longest differential diagnosis, numbering more than 300. Headache is the most common complaint encountered by the primary physician and a staggering 85% of the patients with headache self-medicate. It is estimated that more than 250 million people worldwide have migraine headache only and 50% of population have headache monthly, 15% weekly and 5% daily. More than 90% have unprovoked attack annually and primary headache is the most common type. Some of the most famous personality in the history who suffered from headache are Julius Caesar, Charles Darwin, Alexander—The Great, Ludwig von Beethoven, Rudyard Kipling, Lewis Carroll, etc.

PATHOPHYSIOLOGY

The basic mechanism of transmission of pain is through two types of nerve fibers, namely A delta and C fibers, the former for sharp pain and the later for dull and diffuse pain. The first order neuronal system is situated in the dorsal root ganglion with the ascending sensory pathway, which has three relay stations and three sets of neurons. The second order neuron system cell bodies lies in the dorsal horn of the spinal cord and their axons cross the midline to reach the opposite side, ascending through the spinothalamic tract in the spinal cord and the brainstem to reach the thalamus where the terminal fibers synapse with cells in thalamus. The neurons in the thalamus constitute the third order neuronal system and their axons called thalamocortical fibers, ascending to terminate in the cortex of the parietal lobe where they make synapses with the pain sensing cells of the parietal cortex. Pain sensation of the head and face region are conducted to the parietal lobe through trigeminal root ganglion, which is the seat of the first order neuronal system. The neurons of the trigeminal (gasserian) root ganglion like that of the dorsal root ganglion have distal or peripheral and proximal or central fibers. The second order neuronal system lies in the nucleus of trigeminal nerve situated in the upper three cervical spinal cord segments through the medulla oblongata, pons and mid-brain to terminate in thalamus. The third order neuronal system arises from the thalamic neurons and ascends to terminate again in the parietal lobe. Other than the spinothalamic and trigeminothalamic tract, there is a third ascending sensory pathway called spinoreticulothalamic system. Pain arising from the deeper structures is conducted through this system and is poorly localized. There are also descending sensory fibers from the brainstem that have inhibitory effect on pain, the most important of which is found in the periaqueductal gray matter in the mid-brain. The chemical neurotransmitters for the descending inhibitory pathway are serotonin and noradrenaline in contrast to the ascending pathway that uses acetylcholine.

CLASSIFICATION

The International Headache Society (IHS) rendered first classification in 1988 had three major groups with 14 sections and 220 entities, which were subsequently modified in 2004 to include more conditions that has exceeded more than 300 now. As per the IHS classification (1988), the following 14 groups are:

- Migraine
    - With aura
    - Without aura
- Tension headache
- Cluster headache
- Chronic paroxysmal hemicrania
- Headache unassociated with structural lesion
- Headache due to head trauma
- Headache associated with vascular disorder
- Headache associated with nonvascular intracranial disorder
- Headache associated with substance abuse and withdrawal
- Headache associated with noncephalic infections
- Headache associated with metabolic disorders
- Headache associated with HEENT (Head, Eye, Ear, Nose and Throat) disorders
- Cranial neuralgia and facial pain
- Unclassified/miscellaneous group.

However, for the general practitioner, a better classification system would be primary versus secondary and the main conditions in primary group are migraine, tension headache and cluster headache.

Classification of Migraine (Group 1)

- Migraine without aura (common migraine) code 1.1
- Migraine with aura (classical migraine) code 1.2
- Ophthalmoplegic migraine (code 1.3)
- Retinal migraine (code 1.4)
- Childhood migraine (code 1.5)
- Complicated migraine (code 1.6)
    - Status migrainosus (code 1.6.1)
    - Migrainous infarction (code 1.6.2)
- Migrainous disorder not fulfilling preceding criteria (code 1.7).

Diagnostic Criteria for Migraine

- Five or more attacks of headache lasting for 4 to 72 hours, if untreated
- Any two of the following features:
    - Unilateral headache
    - Pulsating headache
    - Moderate to severe pain intensity
    - Aggravation by exertion
- Nausea with or without vomiting or photophobia or phonophobia
- No evidence of any organic disease.

Diagnostic Criteria for Tension-type Headache

At least 10 previous headache episodes lasting from 30 minutes to 7 days.

- Must have at least two of the following features:
    - Bilateral location
    - Pressing or tightening quality
    - Mild to moderate intensity
    - Not aggravated by routine physical activity
- Absence of the following during headache:
    - Nausea or vomiting
    - Photophobia or phonophobia
- No evidence of organic disease.

Diagnostic Features of Cluster Headache

- Most severe forms of headache
- Unique periodicity
- Autonomic features
- Most common site of pain in trigeminal territory
- Nausea and vomiting rare, unlike in migraine
- Common in males (male to female ratio is 14:1)

- Headache tend to occur during early night (1 to 2 after retiring)
- Attack lasts from 30 minutes to 2 hours
- Patient typically pace the floor unlike lying down in migraine
- 85% are episodic lasting from 2 weeks to 2 months, separated by remissions of 6 months to 1 year
- Psychophysical makeup is like leonine-mouse syndrome (masculine appearance with timid personality).

Diagnostic Criteria or Temporal Arteritis (TA)

As per the American College of Rheumatology, three out of the following criteria should be satisfied for the diagnosis for TA (Giant cell arteritis):

- At least 50 years of age
- New onset of localized headache
- Temporal artery tenderness or decreased pulsation
- ESR at least 50 mm/hr
- Positive histopathology.

Causes of Secondary Headache over 50 Years of Age

- Temporal arteritis
- Intracranial tumors
- Subdural hematoma
- Epidural hematoma
- Cerebrovascular disorders
- Postherpetic neuralgia
- Hypnic headache
- HEENT disorders
- Systemic diseases
- Medication related headache.

Although 90% of the headaches in younger patients are primary, only 66% of those in elderly are primary.

Cranial Neuralgias and Headache with Craniovascular Disorders

The most common cause of cranial neuralgia is trigeminal neuralgia. Other conditions include glossopharyngeal neuralgia, geniculate neuralgia, occipital neuralgia, nasociliary (Charlin) neuralgia, cavernous angiomas, cerebrovascular accident, cerebrovascular thrombosis, saccular aneurysms, dural arteriovenous fistula, etc.

Diagnostic Features of Pseudotumor Cerebri

- 90% patients are young obese women
- Papilledema in 95% of cases

- Headache in 75% cases
- 6th nerve palsy in 25% cases
- Transient visual obstruction in 70% cases
- Increased intracranial pressure (benign intracranial hypertension, more than 20 cm water).

Headache Associated with Sinonasal Disorders

Nose and peripheral nervous system (PNS) disorders are often misdiagnosed as common cause of headache but in reality, only less than 5% of headache are Sinonasal in origin. However, the common causes of sinonasal headache are rhinosinusitis, deviated nasal septum/spurs, concha bullosa, paradoxical turbinate, cysts, polyps, mucocele, and fungal sinusitis, etc.

Causes of Headache Associated with Papilledema

- Intracranial mass (SOL)
- Cerebral venous thrombosis
- Ventricular system obstruction
- Pre-eclampsia and eclampsia
- Meningitis/Encephalitis
- Guillain–Barré syndrome (GBS)
- Head injury
- Optic neuritis
- Central retinal venous thrombosis
- Medications like vitamin A, minocycline, anabolic steroids, etc.
- Meningeal carcinomatosis
- Systemic lupus erythematosus.

Causes of Chronic Progressive Headache in Children and Adolescents

- Neoplasms
  - Medulloblastoma
  - Astrocytoma and glioma
  - Ependymoma
  - Craniopharyngioma
  - Pineal tumors
  - Supratentorial tumors
- Hydrocephalus
- Brain abscess
- Pseudotumor cerebri
- Malformations
  - Arnold-Chiari syndrome
  - Dandy-Walker cyst.

Acute Severe New Onset Headache (First or Worst Headache)

- 20% have subarachnoid hemorrhage (SAH)
- 80% of non-traumatic SAH are due to intracranial saccular aneurysms
- Thunder clap headache may be due to cerebral vasospasms, carotid or vertebral artery dissection, pituitary apoplexy, unruptured intracranial saccular aneurysms or migraine.

Sentinel Headache (Warning Leak)

Before major rupture of a saccular aneurysm, 50% of the patients develop headache and 50% of the major subarachnoid hemorrhage occurs one week within sentinel headache, which is usually of sudden onset. 50% of these patients, who see the doctor, are frequently misdiagnosed. 70% of the cases present with associated symptoms like nausea and vomiting, neck pain and stiffness, blurred or double vision, motor or sensory abnormalities, drowsiness or dizziness and transient loss of consciousness.

Headache Alarms (Red Flags)

These are diagnostic alarms or danger signals alerting to the possibility of an underlying sinister cause needing further investigations. The following features are danger signals or alarms like:

- Headaches occurring after 50 years of age
- Sudden onset of 'first' headache
- Accelerating pattern of headache
- New onset headache in patient with carcinoma or HIV
- Late onset new headache
- Progressively increased headache
- Headache with systemic illness
- Headache with papilledema
- Headache with mental changes
- Focal neurological symptoms and signs.

Practice Guidelines or Indications for CT and MRI in Diagnosis

- Most severe headache ever
- First severe headache over 50 years of age
- Focal neurological sign
- Presence of nuchal rigidity
- Headache worsening under observation
- Onset of headache on exertion
- Decreased alertness or cognition with headache
- Unexplained abnormality of vital signs

- Headache with presence of papilledema
- Headache with cranial nerve palsy.

Diagnostic Roadmap of Headache

The most important approach in the diagnosis of headache is to differentiate between primary and secondary headache. Primary headache is recurrent, benign, without any serious underlying cause or structural disorders and does not cause persistent deficit. More than 90% of the headaches are primary type, which can be diagnosed by proper history taking about the:

- Duration
- Frequency
- Time of onset
- Mode of onset
- Quality
- Site
- Trigger or influencing factor
- Relieving factors
- Radiation
- Any associated symptoms.

The most common form of primary headaches are:

- Migraine
- Tension type of headache
- Cluster headache
- Miscellaneous headache unassociated with any structural lesion.

Secondary headaches account for less than 10% of cases, which are more difficult to diagnose unlike the primary type. A detailed clinical examination and necessary investigations are required for the diagnosis of secondary headache that usually have a underlying cause like meningitis, intracranial hemorrhage and tumor, sinusitis, glaucoma, temporal arteritis, craniofacial neuralgias, psychogenic disorders. A thorough neurological examination should be done whenever required, including dental, ENT and ophthalmological evaluation.

History in Case of Headache

- *Duration:* This is the first guide to know whether the symptoms portraits some malignant or progressive neurological disorder requiring further investigations. Sudden onset of severe headache, possibly followed by impairment of consciousness or focal neurological signs would suggest a serious illness such as subarachnoid hemorrhage or meningitis, whereas patient having headache regularly for many years is likely due to primary headache like migraine or chronic tension type of headache. But headache duration between very acute and chronic type, which has developed over the days, weeks or months may be due to sinusitis, subdural hematoma, cerebral tumor or other case of intracranial tension or temporal arteritis in elderly

- *Frequency:* This is very important in the diagnosis of recurrent headaches in migraine, trigeminal neuralgias, etc. Trigeminal neuralgia headache lasts only for a few seconds, whereas migraine headache recurs one or more times each week and last for a few hours to several days. But cluster headache, which has typical periodicity that usually occurs in bouts, lasting for 2 weeks to 3 months followed by remission to come back again after 3 months to 3 years. Tension type headache has no paroxysmal quality or periodicity in the course, which is persistent throughout for a period with occasional remission
- *Time of onset:* Migraine can start any time of the day or in the early hours of morning, whereas cluster headache has a certain timing that occurs punctually at certain time in the night or day. Tension type headache is present almost throughout the day
- *Mode of onset:* A history of migrainous aura, if present, is diagnostic of migraine. A change of mood, desire for sweets could indicate early warning symptoms of the impending migraine attack. Some of the typical premonitory symptoms are nausea, irritability, increase thirst and hunger, drowsiness, constipation, diarrhea and paresthesias like odd sensation of "pins and needles" or numbness, etc.
- *Site or place of headache:* Unilateral headache are usually due to migraine, cluster headache and trigeminal neuralgia. Migraine often starts in the temporal or occipital region and subsequently progress to evolve one-half or the entire head. But the pain of cluster headache first evolves in the eye and frontal region on one side and could radiate back to occiput or descend to evolve the cheek, teeth, whereas trigeminal neuralgia produces pain in the area of distribution of 2nd and 3rd division of 5th cranial nerve and rarely over the 1st division. The pain in tension type headache is usually bilateral but sometimes could be unilateral especially in patients who have associated migraine
- *Quality and severity:* Most of the time, the quality of the pain is not very specific for differential diagnosis, but throbbing or pulsatile headache is most often associated with vascular headache. Migraine usually starts with a dull headache but may become pulsatile as the intensity increases gradually. Pain in cluster headache is deep, boring and intense whereas in trigeminal neuralgia the pain is like a series of stabs or shock like in nature. Pain in tension type headache is dull, constant, tight and presses like a band around the head. Headache in meningitis or subarachnoid hemorrhage may be very severe. In brain tumor, headache may be mild in initial stage but increases in severity as the tumor grows in size
- *Influencing or aggravating factors:* Vascular headache will be made worse by sudden jarring movements, sneezing, coughing or straining. Light sensitivity is a common feature of diffuse intracranial disturbance like meningitis,

encephalitis and migraine attack also. Menstrual cycle, pregnancy and breastfeeding are known to aggravate headache

- *Precipitating factors:* Triggering factors need to be enquired into every case of headache and avoidance of triggering factors is an important aspect of management of headache. Environmental, social and occupational history should be explored for such possible factors. There should be some specific factors, which may precipitate headache in an individual, which include factors as consumption of cheese, ice cream, tea, coffee, red wine, other dietary items like monosodium glutamate (MSG), etc. Even fatigue, loud sounds, sexual intercourse, emotional changes may be the precipitating factors also
- *Relieving factors:* Pressure on the scalp or use of hot compress is often smoothening in migraine and cluster headache. The severity of tension-type headache is reduced by voluntary relaxation of forehead and jaw muscles and avoidance of jaw clinching. Besides the information on the drugs in treatment, history that might have taken by the patient earlier, the effect of procedures like acupuncture, psychotherapy, yoga, medication and exercises, etc. on the course of treatment, should be also assessed to rationalize the plan of further management
- *Associated symptoms:* Other than premonitory symptoms, headache may be associated like nausea, vomiting, diarrhea, constipation, pain abdomen. Sweating, flushing of skin, running nose, congested and red eyes. History of features like photophobia, phonophobia, taste and smell disturbance should also be enquired.

INVESTIGATIONS

Some of the important investigations that may be required in patients with headache are:

- X-ray sku1l
- X-ray PNS
- X-ray cervical spine and temporomandibular joint (TMJ)
- CSF analysis
- EEG
- CT and MRI, depending on the clinical diagnosis by the treating physician.

It is always desirable before resorting to the latest diagnostic aids like CT, SPECT and MRI, etc. that the general practitioner or physician should first determine the pattern of headache and categorize in a working classification, after taking a detailed history and thorough physical examination.

TREATMENT

There should be a systematic approach for treating headache and drug therapy is the mainstay for such patients. Other than the pharmacological management, psychological therapy and physical therapy are the other components of systematic approach. Very few patients may need surgical intervention and alternative therapies. It is worth noting that almost 70% of the patients attending the headache clinic or general OPD belong to tension type headache. Since most of the patients of headache require analgesics, it is better to avoid narcotic or steroidal analgesic drug because of the risk of developing complications and addictions. It is better to use a single drug initially and later a combination of drug can be tried. The commonly used pharmacological agents for the treatment of headache are:

- NSAIDs (nonsteroidal anti-inflammatory drugs)
- Acetaminophen
- Tramadol
- Opioids like morphine, pentazocine, meperidine, codeine, etc.
- Benzodiazepines
- GABAergic drugs
- Salicylates
- Indomethacin and diclofenac sodium
- Tricyclic antidepressants
- Calcium channel-blockers and beta-blockers
- Serotonins like 5 HT_2 receptor agonist
- Selective 5 HT_1 agonists (triptans)
  - Sumatriptan
  - Eletriptan
  - Zolmitriptan
  - Frovatriptan
  - Naratriptan
  - Almotriptan
  - Rizatriptan.

Drugs Used for Migraine Prophylaxis

- Beta-adrenergic blockers
  - Propranolol (40–120 mg/day)
  - Metoprolol (50–100 mg/day)
  - Atenolol (50–100 mg/day)
  - Nadelol (40–160 mg/day)
- Tricyclic antidepressants
  - Amitriptyline (10–200 mg/day)
  - Nortriptyline (25–75 mg/day)
  - Protriptyline
  - Imipramine
  - Desipramine
  - Doxepin

- Calcium channel blockers
    - Verapamil (80–400 mg)
    - Flunarizine
    - Diltiazem
- 5 HT_2 antagonist
    - Methysergide
    - Cyproheptadine
    - Pizotifen
- NSAIDs
    - Ibuprofen
    - Naproxen
    - Ketoprofen
    - Tolfenamic acid
- GABAergic agonist
    - Valproate
    - Gabapentin
- Miscellaneous
    - Clonidine
    - Dihydroergotamine.

Acute Migraine Specific Drugs

- Sumatriptan (50–200 mg/day)
- Zolmitriptan (5–10 mg/day)
- Naratriptan (2.5–5 mg/day)
- Rizatriptan (10–30 mg/day)
- Eletriptan (40–80 mg/day)
- Almotriptan.

Treatment of Acute Migraine in Children

- NSAIDs
    - Ibuprofen—10 mg/kg (> 4 years)
    - Paracetamol—15 mg/kg (> 4 years)
- Triptans
    - Sumatriptan (> 6 years)
        - Nasal (10 or 20 mg)
        - Oral (50 or 100 mg)
        - Subcutaneous (0.06 mg/kg)
    - Rizatriptan—5 mg (> 12 years)
    - Zolmitriptan—2.5 or 5 mg (> 12 years).

Current Concept in Acute Migraine Treatment

A typical algorithm for treatment of the primary headache disorders should be to: (1) Exclude secondary headache; (2) Diagnose the specific primary disorder; and (3) Chose specific treatment. The mainstream approach to acute migraine treatment is termed as step care or stratified care as per the therapeutic need of the patient starting with simple analgesics and then combinations of analgesics and finally the triptans, depending on the response to the treatment as per the severity of attack, whether mild, moderate, severe or very severe.

Indications of Steroids in Headache Disorders

- Cluster headache
- Temporal arteritis
- Tolosa hunt syndrome
- Costenis syndrome.

Indications of Functional Endoscopic Sinus Surgery (FESS) for Headache in Nose and PNS Disorders

- Septal deviation and spurs
- Concha bullosa
- Paradoxical middle turbinate
- Chronic sinusitis
- Polyps and mucocele
- Mycotic infections
- CSF rhinorrhea.

Treatment of Trigeminal Neuralgia

Out of all the conditions included in IHS classification in the section under craniofacial neuralgia, trigeminal neuralgia is the most common. The most effective pharmacological agent used for this is carbamazepine (tegretol) in the dose of 50–100 mg BID or TID to start with progressive upward titration of the dose up to 1200 mg/day. The other drugs for the condition are clonazepam, baclofen tocainide and anticonvulsants like phenytoin (dilantin), etc.

When medical management is not effective or not tolerated, a series of invasive surgical technique on the trigeminal pathways can be considered, which includes:

- Microvascular compression
- Radiotherapy thermocoagulation of the Gasserian ganglion (Gangliolysis)
- Gamma knife radiosurgery
- Glycerol rhizotomy
- Peripheral branch alcohol injection.

Headache Attributed to Substance or its Withdrawal

Headache induced by acute substance use or exposure as per the international classification for headache disorders are:

- Alcohol-induced headache
- Monosodium glutamate (MSG)-induced headache
- Cocaine-induced headache
- Cannabis-induced headache
- Histamine-induced headache
- Medication overuse headache like opioids, triptans, analgesics, etc.
- Exogenous hormone-induced headache
- Nitric oxide (NO)-induced headache
- Carbon monoxide-induced headache
- Phosphodiesterase (PDE) inhibitor-induced headache
- Calcitonin gene related peptide (CGRP)-induced headache
- Headache attributed to substance withdrawal like caffeine, opioids, etc.

Alternate Therapies for Headache

- Acupuncture
- Biofeedback
- Cognitive behavioral therapy
- Chiropractic (manipulation and massage)
- Aromatherapy
- Herbal medicine
- Hypnotherapy
- Reflexotherapy
- Yoga and meditation
- Osteopathy
- Relaxation therapy.

BIBLIOGRAPHY

1. Bateman ND, Woodford TJ. Facial pain: diagnosis management. CME Bulletin ORL & HNS. 2001;5:50-3.
2. Cussileth BR. The Alternative Medicine Handbook. The Complete Reference Guide to Alternative and Complimentary Therapies. Newyork, Norton. 1998.
3. Evans RW, Mathew NT. Handbook of Headache. Lippincott Williams and Wilkins. 2000.
4. Evans RW. Diagnosis of headaches. "Drugs Today". 1997,33;79-93.
5. Goadby PJ, Oleson J. Diagnostic management of Migraine. British Journal. 1996;312:1279-83.
6. Goadby PJ. Cluster headaches: new perspectives Cephalgia. 1999;19:39-41.
7. http://www.Migrainehelp.com.

8. IHS, Classification and Diagnostic criteria for headache disorders, cranial neuralgias and facial pain. Cephalgia. 1988;8(supp7):1-96.
9. Jones NS. The classification and diagnosis of facial pain. Hospital Medicine. 2001;62: 598-606.
10. Maheshwari MC. Headache: National Book Trust, India. 1994.
11. National Headache Foundation (NHF). http://www/headaches.org.
12. Raskin NH. Headache, 2nd ed. New York: Churchill Livingstone. 1988.
13. Silberstein SD, Goadsby PJ, Lipton RB. Management of migraine, anlogrithmic approach. Neurology. 2000;55:46-52.
14. Silberstein SD, Lipton RB, Goadsby PJ. Headache in Clinical Practice. Martin Duritz. 2002.
15. The International Classification of Headache Disorders, 2nd Edition (1st revision, May 2005).

CHAPTER

7 Anesthetic Considerations in ENT Emergencies

Emergency services are an integral part of any discipline of clinical medicine and are considered as an indicator of the quality of healthcare system. Emergencies pertaining to the ENT specialty can be of varied types ranging from very trivial ones to that of very serious nature like leading to brain abcess. With increasing incidence of road traffic accidents (RTA), industrial and other disasters, the ENT emergencies are on a rise, challenging problems to various specialties of the medical discipline. The anesthesiologist is no exception. Rather the anesthesiologist has an important role in tackling and helping the otorhinolaryngologist in dealing with the situations in mitigating and minimizing the morbidity and mortality.

What are the Common Emergencies Met with

The various emergencies encountered in ENT practice where an anesthesiologist is concerned and frequently called for, includes:

- Foreign bodies
- Infections affecting the airway
- Trauma
- Epistaxis.

PROBLEMS ASSOCIATED WITH ENT EMERGENCIES

- General
  - Hemorrhage
  - Full stomach
  - Shock
  - Sepsis
  - Airway obstruction
- Specific
  - Foreign bodies
  - Infections affecting the airway

- Trauma: Faciomaxillary, laryngeal, nose, ear
  - Faciomaxillary trauma: Airway obstruction, difficult intubation, head injury, cervical cord damage
  - Laryngeal trauma: Air embolism, subcutaneous emphysema
  - Nasal trauma: Upper airway obstruction
  - Aural trauma
- Epistaxis.

Certain Specific Anesthetic Techniques Used in ENT Emergencies

- Cardiopulmonary resuscitation
- Cricothyroidotomy
- Fiberoptic endotracheal intubation
- Awake intubation.

FOREIGN BODIES IN ENT PRACTICE

Foreign Bodies in the Airway

Of all the foreign bodies encountered in ENT practice, the foreign bodies in the airway are the most dangerous and can be a life-threatening emergency. An aspirated solid or semisolid object may lodge in the larynx or trachea. If the object is large enough to cause nearly complete obstruction of the airway, asphyxia may rapidly cause death. Lesser degrees of obstruction or passage of the obstructive object, beyond the carina, can result in less severe signs and symptoms. A foreign body in the airway can lead to a partial obstruction of the airway or a total obstruction. Near-total obstruction of the larynx or trachea can cause immediate asphyxia and death. Since the object pass beyond the carina, its location would depend on the patient's age and physical position at the time of the aspiration. Because the angles made by the main stem bronchi with the trachea are identical until the age of 15 years, foreign bodies are found on either side with equal frequency in persons in this age group. Beyond this age, as the right main bronchus is in a vertical direction in comparison to the left, the aspirated foreign bodies tend to enter the right side rather than the left.

Objects Inhaled

Children are at risk for putting small toys, candies, or nuts into their mouths. Frequently aspirated objects include food (especially nuts and seeds), teeth, dental appliances, etc.

Pathophysiology

The object itself might cause obstruction. Distal to the obstruction, air trapping may occur, leading to local emphysema, atelectasis, hypoxic vasoconstriction, postobstructive pneumonia. Vegetable material may swell over hours or days, worsening the obstruction. Organic foreign bodies, such as oily nuts, induce inflammation and edema. Local inflammation, edema, cellular infiltration, ulceration and granulation tissue formation may contribute to airway obstruction while making bronchoscopic identification and removal of the object more difficult.

Presentation

At times, the patients may be asymptomatic. The original event might have been forgotten. A small number of foreign body aspirations are incidentally found after chest radiography or bronchoscopic inspection. Physical findings may include stridor, fixed wheeze, localized wheeze, or diminished breath sounds.

Choking with severe dyspnea, leading to respiratory or cardiac arrest while eating, might initially be misdiagnosed as myocardial ischemia.

Partial Airway Obstruction

Whenever a foreign body enters the airway, there is an immediate reaction in the form of coughing, gagging or a sensation of choking. The victim exhibits the sign of clutching the throat (universal sign of respiratory obstruction). The initiated cough may not subside until the foreign body gets expelled.

- Stridor—is a noisy inspiration due to turbulent upper airway gas flow. It is frequently seen with airway obstruction and always commands attention. Subclinical stridor (which can be auscultated on the neck with a stethoscope) indicates mild airway compromise. Usually, significant airway compromise must develop before any sign of stridor is evident
- Laryngospasm—is a reflex closure of the upper airway from spasm of the glottic musculature. This form of respiratory obstruction is common in children. It can be due to a foreign body or irritation of the airway due to any cause. If not treated early, it may lead to complete airway obstruction
- Signs and symptoms—they include stridor, inability to speak, pain in the throat, hoarseness, hurried breathing, wheezing, laryngospasm and at times, cyanosis.

Complete Airway Obstruction

Depending on the size of the foreign body, the obstruction may become complete. Complete airway obstruction is a dire medical emergency requiring urgent treatment. Complete obstruction is characterized by inability to talk, weak or no coughing reflex, cyanosis proceeding to unconsciousness. There will not be any breath sounds on auscultation of the chest.

Maneuvers and Treatment Used for Foreign Body Airway Obstruction (FBAO)

The presence of a foreign body and its condition, anatomical location (e.g. larynx, trachea, main lobar or segmental bronchus), shape, composition, position and extent of entrapment by edema or granulation tissue must be identified prior to extraction attempts.

Emergency Methods Used to Relieve Obstruction

These include Heimlich maneuver, back blows and abdominal thrusts.

Bronchoscopy can be used diagnostically and therapeutically. Most aspirated foreign bodies are radiolucent. Radiological procedures do not have extreme diagnostic accuracy and aspiration events are not always detected.

Local inflammation, edema, cellular infiltration, ulceration and granulation tissue formation may contribute to airway obstruction while making bronchoscopic identification and removal of the object more difficult.

The airway becomes more likely to bleed with manipulation; the object is more likely to be obscured and becomes more difficult to dislodge.

Rigid Bronchoscopy

It is the procedure of choice for removing foreign bodies in children and in most adults. It has important advantages over the flexible bronchoscope. The larger diameter of the rigid bronchoscope facilitates the passage of various grasping devices, including a flexible bronchoscope. Suctioning of clotted blood and thick secretions are also better done with this. Another main advantage is that the patient can be ventilated through the rigid scope.

However, the patient has to be heavily sedated or general anesthesia is given for the successful use of this instrument. A jet ventilation device should be available for ventilating the patient during the procedure.

Flexible Bronchoscopy

One of the main advantages of this instrument is that it can be inserted through nose also apart from the oral route. However, the transoral route is preferable, if removal of the foreign body is anticipated. A bite block must be available for using this instrument through this route. Heavy sedation may not always be required to tolerate it. This instrument offers a limited capability to visualize, grasp and remove certain foreign bodies of appropriate size, shape and position as with rigid bronchoscopy. Despite its limitations, use of the flexible fiberoptic bronchoscope may be necessary in patients with maxillofacial or cervical trauma; in whom rigid bronchoscopy is not feasible.

The flexible bronchoscope can provide access to subsegmental bronchi, beyond that provided by the rigid bronchoscope.

Foreign Bodies in the Ear

Foreign bodies can be either in the ear lobe or in the ear canal. Usually, they are more common in children. They can be anything a child can push into his/her ear. They include food items, toys, buttons, small batteries, dangerous things like pins, insects. While playing other children can put some foreign bodies.

Presentation

Many of the foreign bodies may not cause any signs and symptoms unless secondary infection ensues. Other foreign bodies like food and insects can cause redness, pain in the ear or even a discharge from the ear. Hearing may be affected if the object is blocking the ear canal.

Treatment

It includes prompt removal of the foreign body at the earliest opportunity. Organic foreign bodies tend to swell over a period of time making it both difficult and contribute to secondary infection.

Foreign Bodies in the Nose

Children are usually prone for foreign bodies in the nose. They tend to put soft things in the nose. At times, they can lodge in the nose while they are smelling the objects.

Presentation

The usual presentation is in the form of a nasal discharge. The discharge is unilateral and very frequently foul-smelling. Sometimes bleeding from the nose can occur.

Treatment

Treatment is by removal of the foreign body as early as possible. Invariably the child will not cooperate and it is necessary to sedate the child or general anesthesia will very often be required. Anesthetizing a child with an obstructed nostril can be challenging.

Techniques used in removing nasal foreign bodies:

- Positive pressure technique
- Removal by suction catheter
- Grasping the object with an alligator forceps
- Passing a curette beyond foreign body
- Passing a Fogarty catheter beyond, and inflating and removal.

Whatever the technique used, the airway must be protected and appropriate material for managing airway obstruction should be immediately available. Conscious sedation or even general anesthesia may be required in an uncooperative child.

INFECTIONS AFFECTING THE AIRWAY

The infective emergency conditions seen in the emergency room, which are of concern to the anesthesiologist, are invariably that which are closer to the airway, which is always at peril, especially in those which are fulminant.

The various conditions include:

- Peritonsillar abscess
- Retropharyngeal abscess
- Dental abscesses, Ludwig's angina and deep neck abscesses.

Apart from the infections, there is a subset class of abnormal masses or growths in close proximity of the airways, which may compromise the airway leading to an emergency situation. Some of the conditions that are encountered include:

- Cellulitis of the neck
- Neck and upper airway masses.

These include hemangioma, lymphangioma, branchial cleft cyst (infants), reactive lymphadenopathy, branchial cleft cyst, thyroglossal duct cyst (children and young adults), salivary gland or parotid neoplasm, oral cavity neoplasms, metastatic carcinomas, lymphomas, thyroid disorders (adults), etc.

- Angioedema of the upper airway
- Uvular edema.

The prime concern in most of the above conditions is maintenance of an adequate and patent airway. The infectious conditions can lead to sepsis in addition and the abscesses likely to burst leading to septicemia apart from the obstruction. The various inflammatory conditions or the malignancies can fragment or cause bleeding into the airway.

Peritonsillar Abscess

It is the most commonly occurring deep space infection of the head and neck. It is the collection of purulent material between the tonsillar capsule and the superior constrictor and palatopharyngeus muscle. It is most common in second and third decades of life.

Complications

Complications of this condition include airway obstruction, rupture of abscess leading to aspiration, epiglottitis, septicemia, cavernous sinus thrombosis, retropharyngeal abscess, mediastinitis, etc. Most of the complications can present themselves as an emergency in adults.

Anesthetic Implications

Airway maintenance, management of infection and septicemia, shock can be challenging. Extreme care should be taken while inducing anesthesia, intubation of the patient. Airway compromise can be accentuated while induction. There is every chance of the abscess getting ruptured while intubating. Successful achievement of airway can be the key for successful conduct of anesthesia.

Retropharyngeal Abscess

This extends from the base of the skull to the tracheal bifurcation. In children, retropharyngeal abscess, usually, are suppurative changes within a lymph node, whereas in adults, it is the direct extension of purulent debris from an adjacent site, such as Ludwig's angina. Therefore, retropharyngeal abscess in an adult is more likely to extend into the mediastinum.

Complications

Catastrophic complications include extension of infection to the mediastinum, upper airway asphyxia from direct pressure or sudden rupture of the abscess.

Anesthetic Implications

Intravenous hydration and antibiotic treatment should be started in the emergency department (ED) itself, before the patient can be brought to the operating theater (OT). Although few patients can be managed with intravenous antibiotics, most patients will require surgical intervention. The anesthetic considerations are similar to that of peritonsillar abscess.

Dental Abscesses, Ludwig's Angina and Deep Neck Abscesses

A dental abscess may spread into the sublingual and submandibular spaces. Thus, they may cause marked floor of the mouth edema. The implications for the anesthesiologist include, trismus, difficult laryngoscopy among others.

Ludwig's angina is an infection of the submental, sublingual and submandibular spaces causing elevation and posterior displacement of the tongue. The implications include poor dental hygiene, dysphagia, trismus, odynophagia, edema of the upper midline neck and marked edema of the floor of the mouth. Airway compromise should be of prime concern in these patients. Many of the patients with Ludwig's angina will require awake fiberoptic intubation or awake tracheostomy.

Angioedema of the Upper Airway

It is a nondemarcated swelling of dermal or submucosal layers of the skin and mucosa. It is usually nonpruritic but can be painful. It can have a sudden onset and rapid progression.

Anesthetic Implications

Intravenous access should be established and airway examined with fiberoptic nasopharyngoscopy as soon as possible. Patients with life-threatening edema should undergo fiberoptic intubation with preparation for an emergent surgical airway. Other emergency measures like epinephrine, antihistaminics, and corticosteroids should be administered as indicated according to the situation. Airway patency and establishment take utmost priority.

TRAUMA EMERGENCIES IN ENT PRACTICE

By definition, the trauma patient should be considered to have at least a potentially difficult airway.

Establishment of Airway in Trauma

Airway management in the trauma patient poses several unique challenges. Success requires excellent assessment skills, an understanding of the physiology of injury, a thorough knowledge of airway pharmacology.

Things to be looked for in trauma airway management:

- Disrupted airway anatomy
- Cervical spine injury
- Shock
- Chest trauma
- Traumatic brain injury (TBI).

Disrupted Airway Anatomy

In cases of distorted anatomy, the approach must be one that minimizes the potential for catastrophic deterioration. Waiting for the nearly obstructed airway to become completely obstructed can be disastrous. The optimal approach for airway management will vary, depending on the clinical scenario. In patients with signs of significant airway compromise (e.g. stridor, drooling, respiratory distress, expanding neck hematoma), the risk of using neuromuscular blockade is high and it may be most appropriate to attempt awake intubation with sedation or proceed directly to a surgical airway. When symptoms are modest but elective intubation is still indicated (e.g. before interfacility transport), a combined approach may be used, in which an awake technique is used to ensure adequacy of laryngoscopy; then rapid sequence intubation (RSI) is used for the actual intubation. This can be accomplished by gentle laryngoscopy or nasopharyngoscopy.

Cervical Spine Injury

All severely injured blunt trauma patients should be assumed to have a cervical spine injury until and otherwise proved. In many instances, the cervical spine might have been immobilized by the prehospital caregivers. This, even though, is required to prevent further injury, can cause problems.

If urgent airway management is needed, do not waste time getting a cross-table lateral cervical spine X-ray prior to intubation. Instead, assume all patients have cervical injury and maintain in line stabilization at all times. Although no definitive study has demonstrated the safety of oral intubation in the presence of cervical spine injury, an increasing body of literature argues in favor of the safety of this maneuver. Several large series and one cinefluoroscopic study show no evidence that properly performed RSI with in line cervical immobilization presents any hazard to the patient, even in the presence of proven cervical spine injury.

Shock

Patients suffering significant injury may have obvious or occult hypotension from many different sources. Victims of blunt multisystem trauma are especially vulnerable. Shock in this patient population can be broadly classified as hemorrhagic (e.g. external, intrathoracic, intra-abdominal, retroperitoneal, long bone) or nonhemorrhagic (e.g. tension pneumothorax, pericardial tamponade, myocardial contusion, spinal shock). A diligent search for the primary source (s) of hypotension must begin at once. Remember that, patients on the verge of cardiovascular collapse often maintain a "normal" blood pressure, especially if they are young.

Chest Trauma

Chest injury results from a variety of conditions and impairs ventilation and oxygenation. These conditions include pneumothorax, hemothorax, flail chest, pulmonary contusion and open chest wounds. As far as practicable, patients with a known or suspected pneumothorax should have tube thoracostomy performed before intubating. Insertion of the chest tube may restore hemodynamic stability and oxygenation, thus making the intubation safer.

Traumatic Brain Injury

In the patient with traumatic brain injury and impaired cerebral autoregulation, stimulation of the airway during laryngoscopy may worsen intracranial hypertension. Rapid Sequence Intubation (RSI) is the procedure of choice for airway control in the brain-injured patient. The technique should be focused on methods to attenuate the potential rise in ICP that accompanies laryngoscopic examination. Drugs like lidocaine may be used to attenuate this physiological response. Fentanyl attenuates the indirect response and should also be considered, provided the patient is hemodynamically stable. Etomidate, a drug that protects the brain while maintaining stable hemodynamics, is the preferred induction agent.

Assessment of Airway

During the primary survey, one should immediately assess for:

- Injury to the face, mouth, or neck that may make the process of intubation difficult or impossible
- The potential for cervical spine injury and the need for in line cervical stabilization
- Chest injury that may limit the patient's respiratory reserve
- Signs of obvious or occult hemodynamic instability that can be worsened or unmasked by some of the pharmacologic agents used for rapid sequence intubation (RSI)

- The presence of traumatic brain injury, which may alter airway management decision, making and drug selection.

Intubation

In most busy emergency departments, a sizable number of intubations are performed on patients suffering from major trauma.

Points to Remember in Trauma Patients

- Rapid bedside assessment helps in anticipating difficult airway
- Always look for cervical spine injury, occult hypovolemia, traumatic brain injury, etc.
- In line stabilization of the neck will prevent further cervical ford injury
- Always maintain adequate CNS perfusion and oxygenation at all costs in a patient with traumatic brain injury
- Many of the drugs used for rapid sequence intubation (RSI) may precipitate hypotension in the hypovolemic patient
- Oral intubation, using RSI, is the method of choice in most trauma patients
- Always have an individualized plan for airway management in trauma patients.

Faciomaxillary Trauma

Trauma to the face can present in any combination of soft tissue contusions, lacerations, maxillofacial fractures and dental damage. The most common mechanism of injury is falls. Sporting injuries, fights and motor vehicle collusions account for the rest. Injury to the maxillary central incisors accounts for 70% dental injuries. Management of dentoalveolar trauma depends on the extent of tooth and alveolar involvement, the degree of development of the tooth and the age of the patient. Since more than 50% of all maxillofacial injuries are due to motor vehicle accidents, they may be also associated with injuries to the chest, abdomen, head injury and injury to the long bones as well.

Implications for the Anesthesiologist

Maintenance of the Airway

The airway may be potentially or actually compromised by blood, avulsed teeth, dentures, bone pieces or foreign bodies. The tongue may become swollen due to edema or hematoma or its motion may be uncontrollable due to unstable mandibular fractures. The possibility of direct laryngeal injury should always be kept in mind in these type of injuries. Airway obstruction may supervene when impaired consciousness results due to head injury or shock secondary or excessive blood loss.

Control of Bleeding

Hemorrhage should always be controlled. Replacement of lost blood is also of prime concern. Aspiration of blood clots may present a further problem. Endotracheal intubation may be difficult due to presence of blood.

Gastric Emptying

Due to the injury or other causes, gastric emptying may be delayed and hence, all these type of patients should be assumed to have full stomach.

Nasal Fracture

Any significant central midface trauma should be considered highly suspicious of a nasal bone fracture. A direct impact is most likely to cause a fracture, because there is no soft tissue to dissipate the force. In younger patients, the bones are denser and more elastic, whereas in older patients, the bones are less dense and more brittle. The diagnosis of nasal fracture is clinical. Swelling, tenderness, crepitance, ecchymosis or nasal deformity indicate its occurrence.

Complications of Nasal Fracture

These include nasal deformity, deviated nasal septum, septal hematoma, cribriform plate fracture and associated facial, head or spinal injuries. Fracture through the cribriform plate is associated with a cerebrospinal fluid (CSF) leakage. CSF rhinorrhea is suspected when there is a clear nasal discharge following facial injury.

Anesthetic Implications

Associated head injuries and cervical spine injury should always be ruled out or taken into consideration while anesthetizing for nasal fractures. Associated facio-maxillary trauma can pose a problem while establishing an airway.

Laryngeal Trauma

External laryngeal trauma is a rare but potentially dangerous injury coming to the emergency room. Blunt trauma to the larynx occurs primarily as a result of motor vehicle accidents, personal assaults, or sports injuries.

The signs and symptoms include hoarseness, anterior neck into palpation, dyspnea, stridor, cough, dysphagia and or hemoptysis. With more significant or worsening injury pain, dyspnea or cough develops and subcutaneous emphysema may become evident.

Anesthetic Implications

The two primary goals in the management of acute laryngeal trauma are preservation of life by maintaining airway and restoration of function. If the lumen of the laryngeal airway is compromised by ecchymosis and edema but no gross disruption and the tracheal lumen can be identified, it may be secured by intubation or with an endotracheal tube advanced over a flexible bronchoscope. If the laryngeal lumen cannot be visualized because of gross anatomical disruption or edema and hemorrhage, urgent tracheostomy is the preferred method of airway control.

EPISTAXIS IN ENT PRACTICE

Because the blood supply of the nasal mucosa ultimately originates from the carotid arteries, acute epistaxis is potentially serious, especially if the patient is frail or elderly. Most of the epistaxis cases are self-limited and can be managed conservatively.

Epistaxis has an increased incidence during the dry, colder winter months. The duration, severity of the hemorrhage and the site of initial bleeding are the markers for the diagnosis and treatment of epistaxis. Inquire about previous epistaxis, hypertension, hepatic or other systemic disease, family history, easy bruising, or prolonged bleeding after minor surgical procedures. Recurrent episodes of epistaxis, even if self-limited, should raise suspicion for significant nasal pathology. It can be anterior or posterior epistaxis.

Anterior Epistaxis

This represents 90% of all nose bleeds, with the majority originating from the Kiesselbach's plexus. It is common in children. The most common cause is idiopathic or related to upper respiratory infections.

The treatment includes direct pressure, vasoconstrictive agents, nasal packing and cautery.

Posterior Epistaxis

It is far less common than anterior epistaxis. It is more common in the elderly and is believed to be due to arteriosclerosis of the large posterior nasal cavity vessels. The most common site of bleeding is posterior to inferior turbinates, about 6 to 7.5 cm posterior to the vestibule. Typically, the bleeding is more profuse than anterior epistaxis and may be more difficult to control.

The treatment is posterior nasal packing. Direct pressure is ineffective. Blind attempts at chemical, heat or electrocautery can cause injury and more bleeding. Significant or uncontrolled bleeding from a posterior site may require operative management; this occurs in about 30% of the cases.

Anesthetic Considerations

As the bleeding, especially the posterior bleed, is likely to be more profuse and difficult to control, it is necessary to establish an IV line, blood grouping and cross-matching and coagulation studies wherever required. Whenever packing is done, close observation of the patient is necessary to identify the danger of pack dislodge and also further bleeding.

As always, first address the ABCs (airway, breathing, and circulation). Rarely, severe epistaxis may necessitate endotracheal intubation. Hemodynamic instability should take precedence over obtaining a lengthy history.

A significant reduction of elevated blood pressure can usually be obtained with analgesia and mild sedation alone.

Posterior nasal packing is particularly uncomfortable for the patient and promotes hypoxia and hypoventilation. Failure to admit and appropriately monitor all patients who require posterior packing may result in significant mortality. Elderly patients or patients with cardiac disorders or chronic obstructive pulmonary disease (COPD) should receive supplemental oxygen.

Other Hemorrhagic Conditions in ENT Emergencies

Post-tonsillectomy Bleeding

Postoperative bleeding is a well-known complication of tonsillectomy that can lead to death either from airway obstruction or hemorrhagic shock.

The incidence ranges from 1 to 6%, with approximately 50% requiring surgical intervention. There is a significantly higher incidence of bleeding in patients between 21 and 30 years of age and hemorrhage is less common in children under the age of 6. Although bleeding can be seen within 24 hours of surgery, most hemorrhage occur between days 5 and 10.

Anesthetic Implications

This can be fatal and requires prompt intervention with control of airway. The patient requires to be nil per oral (NPO), monitoring with pulse oximetry and kept upright. Immediate IV access is required, blood drawn for CBC, coagulation studies, blood grouping and cross matching.

Massive bleeding is rare, but if occurs, intubation may be the only means of protecting the airway. This is always difficult as there can be oropharyngeal edema from recent surgery and blood obscuring visualization of the cords. Plans should be made for an emergent cricothyrotomy, prior to attempting intubation.

SPECIFIC ANESTHETIC TECHNIQUES USED IN ENT EMERGENCIES

Cardiopulmonary Resuscitation

The first and foremost objective of treatment in any emergency situation including ENT emergencies is to see whether the patient requires resuscitation or in other words, treat if there is cardiac arrest. The ABC algorithm should and must be done by any physician attending on the patient.

The actions taken during the first few minutes of an emergency are critical to victim survival. Basic Life Support (BLS) defines this sequence of actions and saves lives. The BLS includes:

- Prompt recognition and action for myocardial infarction and stroke to prevent respiratory and cardiac arrest
- Rescue breathing for victims of respiratory arrest
- Chest compressions and rescue breathing for victims of cardiopulmonary arrest
- Attempted defibrillation of patients with ventricular fibrillation (VF) or ventricular tachycardia (VT) with an automated external defibrillator (AED)
- Recognition and relief of FBAO.

Early CPR is the best treatment for cardiac arrest until the arrival of AED and advanced cardiovascular life support (ACLS).

How Early CPR Helps

Early CPR prevents VF from deteriorating to asystole, may increase the chance of defibrillation, contributes to preservation of heart and brain function and significantly improves survival. Early defibrillation is the single greatest determinant of survival for adult victims of cardiac arrest.

Public access defibrillation (PAD) is a health care initiative to make AED's available throughout the community, for use by trained laypersons. PAD holds promise to be the single greatest advance in the treatment of VF arrest, since the development of CPR. PAD programs have achieved resuscitation success rates as high as 49%.

The entire resuscitation process can be divided into three distinctive phases. They are basic life support (BLS), advanced cardiac life support (ACLS) and prolonged life support.

Three BLS actions; early access, early CPR and early defibrillation—serve as the foundation for emergency cardiovascular care throughout the community. Each community should identify weaknesses in its chain of survival and strengthen the chain through CPR training programs, effective PAD initiatives and an optimized EMS.

Foreign Body Airway Obstruction (FBAO)

Foreign body airway obstruction is a relatively uncommon but preventable cause of cardiac arrest. This form of death is much less common than death caused by other emergencies.

The FBAO is not a common problem among submersion/near drowning victims. Water does not act as a foreign body and does not obstruct the airway. Near drowning victims require immediate provision of CPR, particularly rescue breathing, to correct hypoxia.

The FBAO should be considered as a cause of deterioration in any victim, especially a younger victim, who suddenly stops breathing, becomes cyanotic and falls unconscious for no apparent reason. FBAO in adults, usually, occurs during eating. Elderly patients with dysphagia are also at risk for FBAO and should take care while drinking or eating.

Recognition of FBAO

Because recognition of airway obstruction is the key to successful outcome, it is important to distinguish this emergency from fainting, stroke, heart attack, seizure, drug overdose or other conditions that may cause sudden respiratory failure but requires different treatment. Foreign bodies may cause either partial or complete obstruction.

Partial Airway Obstruction

This can be recognized by noisy airflow, which may also be accompanied by retraction. Snoring suggests that the partial obstruction is hypopharyngeal, due to the base of tongue. Crowing suggests that there is laryngospasm, gurgling points to the presence of foreign matter and wheezing signals bronchial obstruction. With partial obstruction, the victim may be capable of either "good air exchange" or "poor air exchange".

With good air exchange, the victim is responsive and can cough forcefully, although frequently, there is wheezing in between the coughs. As long as good air exchange occurs, the victim can be encouraged to spontaneous coughing and breathing efforts. At this point, the rescuer should not interfere with the victim's own attempts to expel the foreign body but should stay with the victim and monitor these attempts. If partial obstruction persists, emergency medical services (EMS) can be activated.

Signs of poor air exchange include a weak and ineffective cough, high-pitched noise while inhaling, increased respiratory difficulty and possibly cyanosis.

The victim with FBAO may immediately demonstrate poor air exchange or may demonstrate initially good exchange that progresses to poor air exchange. Treat a victim with partial obstruction and poor air exchange as if he had a complete airway obstruction and act immediately.

Complete Airway Obstruction

Complete airway obstruction is an emergency that will result in death within minutes, if not treated. This is recognized when one cannot hear or feel airflow at the mouth or nose. When there are spontaneous breathing movements, the presence of inspiratory retraction of supraclavicular and intercostal areas and absent chest expansion with inhalations, provide additional clues. During apnea, complete airway obstruction is recognized by the difficulty encountered to inflate the lungs when attempting to ventilate the patient.

The immediate sequelae of airway obstruction can also be suspected on clinical grounds. Hypercarbia, for example, is suspected when there is somnolence and is confirmed by measurement of blood gases. Hypoxemia is suspected when there is tachycardia, restlessness, sweating or cyanosis and is confirmed by measurement of arterial blood gases. Absence of cyanosis, however, does not rule out severe hypoxemia. During acute airway obstruction, attempts at clearing the airway and reoxygenation have absolute priority over arterial blood gas determinations.

Methods of Removal of Foreign Body

Several techniques are used throughout the world to relieve FBAO and it is difficult to compare the effectiveness of any one method with the other. Most resuscitation councils recommend one or more of the following:

- The Heimlich abdominal thrusts
- Back blows
- Chest thrusts.

The Heimlich Maneuver

This is also known as sub-diaphragmatic abdominal thrusts or abdominal thrusts. This is recommended for lay rescuer relief of FBAO in responsive adult (~ 8 years age) and child (1 to 8 years) victims in many countries. It is not recommended for relief of FBAO in infants. The Heimlich maneuver is also recommended by the American Heart Association (AHA) and several other resuscitation councils for use by healthcare providers for unresponsive adult and child (but not infants) victims.

Some resuscitation councils recommend that the rescuer provide up to 5 backblows/slaps as the initial maneuver, with the back slaps delivered between the shoulder blades with the heel of the rescuer's hand. If back slaps fail, up to 5 abdominal thrusts are then attempted and groups of back slaps and abdominal thrusts are repeated.

The Heimlich abdominal thrusts elevate the diaphragm and increase airway pressure, forcing air from the lungs. This may be sufficient to create an artificial cough and expel a foreign body from the airway. Abdominal thrusts, however, may cause complications. For this reason, the Heimlich maneuver should never be performed unless it is necessary. Reported complications of this maneuver include damage to the internal organs, such as rupture or laceration of abdominal or thoracic viscera. In fact, victims who receive Heimlich maneuver should be medically evaluated to rule out any life-threatening complications. To minimize the complications, do not place your hands on the xiphoid process of sternum or on the lower margins of the rib cage. Your hands should be below this area but above the navel in the midline. Some complications can occur even if the Heimlich maneuver is performed correctly. Regurgitation may occur as a result of abdominal thrusts and may be associated with aspiration.

Advanced Cardiac Life Support (ACLS)

The main aim of advanced cardiac life support is to establish the spontaneous circulation of the patient. It consists of establishment of an intravenous (IV) access, administration of drugs like vasopressors, antiarrhythmics, atropine, sodium bicarbonate, calcium chloride, etc.

Prolonged Life Support

This support for a victim of cardiac arrest is given in the ICU's of a hospital. The main aim of this phase of resuscitation is that of cerebral resuscitation. This consists of support of the various physiological systems (respiratory, cardiovascular, renal, cerebral, etc). This phase starts, once the patient is stabilized with his/her own spontaneous circulation and shifted to the hospital.

CRICOTHYROIDOTOMY

It is performed to establish an emergency airway in a patient with upper airway obstruction when endotracheal intubation is impossible or contraindicated. It is used as a temporary measure until more definitive airway control such as an unhurried tracheostomy can be accomplished.

Technique

- A 14 or 16 gauge catheter with needle obturator is inserted in the midline percutaneously, at an angle and directed caudally through the cricothyroid membrane
- The needle is withdrawn upon tracheal entry and the plastic cannula secured with tape
- If available, a cricothyroidotomy cannula may be inserted
- Ventilation may be accomplished by connecting the catheter to a high pressure source of oxygen or a jet ventilator
- Alternately, the catheter may be attached to a self-inflating resuscitation bag or anesthesia machine
  - An adapter from a 7.5 or 8 mm endotracheal tube fitted tightly into the barrel of a 3 mL disposable syringe without the plunger
  - A 7 mm endotracheal tube fitted inside a 5 mL syringe and cuff inflated
- The application of 30 cm H_2O pressure can provide a flow of 5 L/min through a 14 gauge needle.

AWAKE INTUBATION

Awake intubation techniques comprise all techniques in which consciousness is intentionally maintained during the intubation. This is to be distinguished from the practice of administering sedating drugs in lieu of neuromuscular blocking agents, to facilitate unconscious intubation. The three most common of these awake techniques are blind nasotracheal intubation, awake oral intubation, and fiberoptic intubation.

Awake Blind Nasotracheal Intubation

It is rapidly being supplanted by superior techniques of oral intubation with neuromuscular blockade, even in the prehospital setting. The nasotracheal technique takes longer, has a higher failure rate, has a higher complication rate, and requires smaller tube sizes than rapid sequence oral intubation. It is likely that in the one remaining indication for nasotracheal intubation may be the patient with a difficult airway who is breathing spontaneously and for whom rapid sequence intubation (RSI) may not be advisable.

Awake Oral Intubation

In this technique, a sedative agent is administered, liberal airway anesthesia is provided and the patient is intubated orally, with a laryngoscope, "awake". In this context, awake means that the patient can follow simple instructions, provide feedback to the operator and respond to what is happening. The classic context for awake intubation is the patient with distorted upper-airway anatomy, such as that resulting from blunt or penetrating anterior neck trauma, who requires intubation.

Technique

- Prepare the patient. Ensure that the patient is well-oxygenated and that the procedure has been explained to the greatest extent possible to alleviate fear and facilitate cooperation. Assemble all necessary equipment
- Anesthetize the airway. The standard method is to spray the mouth, tongue, oropharynx and larynx with lidocaine spray using a laryngeal spray device. This requires a little patience and compassion but is extremely effective
- Sedate the patient. This is usually done just before, or at the same time as, the topical anesthesia, depending on the method and agents chosen. A good choice would be 1 to 2 mg of midazolam, accompanied by 50 to 100 μg of fentanyl (for analgesia) if desired. Both of these drugs require 3 to 5 minutes to demonstrate peak effects, so the timing of the sedation, anesthesia and intubation is important. Titration is necessary
- Perform the laryngoscopy. Talk to the patient, depending on the level of consciousness; gently advance the laryngoscope to where the cords can be visualized. The patient should be obtunded but breathing spontaneously throughout. At this point, the endotracheal tube (ETT) can be inserted, or more potent agents, such as neuromuscular blocking agents, and additional sedation, can be administered, followed by intubation, if desired. Visualization of the cords with laryngoscopy demonstrates the adequacy of the approach

and may permit the administration of neuromuscular blocking agents if this is considered desirable. Whether to intubate immediately or defer for later and a controlled RSI will depend on the potential for progressively increased airway difficulty. One might elect to immediately intubate an airway bum or anaphylaxis with progressive swelling, whereas a patient with a stable anatomic picture, being intubated for another reason such as head injury, might be better served by deferring shortly for a controlled RSI

- Consider the need for additional sedation. Also, as with all intubations in the emergency department, independent confirmation of tube placement and a chest radiograph are mandatory.

FIBEROPTIC ENDOTRACHEAL INTUBATION

This skill is an important one for the emergency physician, both to facilitate endotracheal intubation of the difficult airway and to perform diagnostic and therapeutic procedures on the upper airway. Few emergency physicians and emergency departments are equipped for this procedure. This procedure is an invaluable technique in airway management, particularly in patients in which standard laryngoscopy and orotracheal intubation have failed or are anticipated to be difficult or impossible.

The scope should be of sufficient caliber and stiffness to allow intubation over itself without kinking, while at the same time, maintaining flexibility and ease of manipulation. A 4 to 4.5 mm outside-diameter (OD) fiberoptic scope is best. The scope should be of sufficient length (60 cm) to allow bronchoscopy and airway toilet in the Emergency department (ED). A separate channel for the insufflation of oxygen, the injection of local anesthetic or saline, and suctioning is essential.

This technique is best suited for predicted difficult intubation, where C-spine immobility required, anatomic abnormalities, failed intubation in the "cannot intubate, can oxygenate" scenarios.

Success depends on familiarity and skill in using the device and on patient selection and setting. The single study looking at fiberoptic intubation in the ED, identified a 70% success rate after gaining some experience. In the hands of trained endoscopists, the success rate approaches 100%. Patient complications with this technique are uncommon and include mucosal damage to the airway and epistaxis. As with all techniques, damage to the vocal apparatus is possible but rare. The most frequent complication is damage to the scope from biting, twisting, kinking, or dropping the scope.

Contraindications of Fiberoptic Intubation

- Excessive secretions, blood in the airway
- Upper airway obstruction due to foreign bodies or other lesions
- Inadequate oxygenation by bag and mask because of time required.

Precautions to be taken while using the scope:

- Do not drop the scope
- Use a bite block to protect the scope
- Avoid acute bending and kinking of the scope
- Lubricate the scope adequately
- Do not flex the tip against undue resistance or use it to move tissue out of the way
- Clean the working channel immediately after use.

Technique of Intubation

It is always better to use it on mannequins before managing it in the ED.

- Gather all the equipments required (topical airway anesthetics, proper endotracheal tubes, biteblocks, lubricants, suction apparatus, additional airway equipments, etc.)
- Obtain an able assistant
- Prepare the patient—explaining the procedure, antisialogogue, IV line establishment, topically anesthestizing the airway
- Lubricate the tube and slide it over the scope, up to the handle of the scope
- Put a drop of silicone liquid on the tip of the scope to prevent fogging
- Put in the bite block, if the oral route is chosen
- Stand up straight at the head end of the bed. Keep the scope in the midline. Use the thumb to toggle the tip, control lever up and down
- The base of the tongue is "up", advance slowly while flexing the tip up to pass over the back of the tongue; the epiglottis comes into view; keep it above you; the pearly white cords come into view opening and closing with respiration; advance the scope in between the cords during inspiration
- Once inside the trachea, advance the scope so that the carina is seen
- Now advance the tube and the scope slowly into the trachea
- Once in trachea, slowly withdraw the scope out of the airway
- Confirm the position of the endotracheal tube.

Airway Management in the Prehospital Setting

The principles of prehospital airway management are mostly similar to those of management in the ED. Limited equipment, availability or non-availability of appropriate drugs, necessary expertise, transport considerations, etc. however, hinders the procedure of endotracheal intubation in the prehospital management of the airway.

A quick evaluation of the patient, with particular focus on the assessment of the airway and ventilation should always be done in the field.

Intubation in the Prehospital Period

It is of utmost importance to note whether the patient is maintaining the airway, ventilating and oxygenating adequately and protecting his/her airway to decide the requirement of endotracheal intubation in this setting.

Obstructed airway, noisy breathing, deep coma with unresponsiveness, apnea are some observations indicating inadequacy of maintaining the airway. Airway repositioning by head tilt, chin lift and jaw thrust maneuvers can help in the management.

Absence of airway reflexes like gagging, coughing, vomiting indicate that the patient may have inadequacy of protecting the airway from aspiration of gastric contents. Aspiration of stomach contents is a serious adverse event and must be prevented.

The next step is to oversee the oxygenation and ventilation adequacy. If in doubt, either administration of oxygen, bag-mask ventilation should always be instituted at the earliest.

If it becomes necessary to intubate, the best method should be selected depending on the patients circumstances, equipments and facilities available, experience of the intubator, etc.

Points to Remember

- Always weigh the risks and benefits of intubation in the prehospital setting against transport to the ED. In many circumstances, rapid transport might be the best way of managing the airway.
- There are very few airway emergencies in the prehospital setting that will not be managed with proper bag-mask ventilation until the patient can be transported to the hospital.
- Newer devices such as a laryngeal mask airway (LMA), combitube may have a role in prehospital care of the patients.

BIBLIOGRAPHY

1. Adams AP, Hermit PB, Rogers MC, Wedley JR. Emergency Anaesthesia. Facio-maxillary, Ear, Nose and Throat problems. Edward Arnold (Publishers) Ltd. 1986;pp.154-63.
2. Airway foreign bodies: google.com/site/drtbalusotolaryngologylHome.
3. Donegan JH. Manual of anesthesia for emergency surgery. In: anesthesia for Emergency Otolaryngologic and Facial Surgery. Asiddao CB (Ed). Churchill Livingstone. 1987;pp. 39-56.
4. Somnath S, et al. Emergency otrhinolaryngological cases in medical college, Kolkata - A statistical analysis.
5. Tintinalli JE. Emergency Medicine: A Comprehensive Study Guide, 6th edition; McGraw-Hill publications. 2003;1464-500.
6. Walls RM, et al. Manual of Emergency Airway Management. 2000.
7. Warshawsky ME. The diagnosis and treatment of foreign bodies in the airway are a challenge for otolaryngologists an overview. emedicine.medscape.com/article/872498.

CHAPTER

8 Pharyngeal and Esophageal Foreign Body

Foreign body in upper food passages is a common emergency in ENT practice. Any object, which is retained in the pharynx or esophagus, is a foreign body. Foreign body can be defined as a substance either exogenous or endogenous found in the body, where it is not present anatomically.

ETIOLOGY

Age

- Children: Foreign bodies are commonly ingested by small children. Children tend to place and explore most objects in their mouth and there is significant risk of foreign body ingestion. Poor children, who are not given individual attention and who are left to feed themselves at an early age, are more liable to swallow foreign body
- Old age: The incidence of foreign body (FB) rises in old people, who get lumps of meat impacted in esophagus; this may be due to the lack of propulsion efficiency or to the fact that patient is often edentulous and unable to masticate his food properly. Tough meat, if improperly chewed, may get impacted
- Dental factor: A patient who has artificial denture, is unable to detect a fish or meat bone in the mouth as easily as a person with a normal palate, is therefore, more likely to swallow a foreign body. If the denture or palate is ill, fitting or broken, it may itself be swallowed and this occasionally occurs, while the patient is drunk or asleep.

Esophageal Factor

A stricture of the esophagus is more likely to occlude the passage of a small foreign body, which would normally pass through. In a carcinomatous stricture, the first sign is lodging of a foreign body, with the sudden onset of dysphagia or even aphagia.

Type of Food

Carelessness in the preparation of food is a factor in the lodging of a foreign body. Certain types of food are eaten very rapidly because the patient does not suspect the presence of bones. Stews and soups may contain meat with splinters of bone attached. Fish cakes, fish fingers may also contain bones, which may become impacted in the alimentary tract.

Voluntary Swallowing

Foreign bodies are swallowed voluntarily by patients who attempt suicide.[1] Occasionally, bizarre ingested foreign bodies, sometimes multiple, are found in psychologically disturbed, mentally retarded and prisoners.[2]

Altered Sensorium

Reduced protective reflexes, for example, drugs, alcohol, etc.

TYPES OF FOREIGN BODIES

Sharp or Blunt

Sharp ones tend to lodge in any part of pharynx or esophagus, small fish or meat bones are the commonly encountered foreign bodies in the pharynx. This may get lodged in the tonsil, vallecula, base of tongue and pyriform fossa. Coins and disc-shaped objects that pass through the mouth and pharynx of a child may then lodge in upper part of esophagus. Open safety pins stay in the esophagus because of the resilience of the pin when the point is uppermost or by penetration of the esophageal wall when the point is downwards.[1]

Battery Ingestion

Almost every household contains several items operated by miniature batteries. The disc batteries are encountered in watches, clocks, calculators, games, toys and in hearing aids. A battery lodged in the esophagus poses a severe hazard from caustic damage. Leakage of caustic alkaline results in tissue liquefaction and it can culminate in an esophageal perforation after several hours.[2]

Foreign Body can be Radiopaque or Radiolucent

- Radiopaque FB's are bones, chicken, meat and metallic FB. Common metallic FB are coins, pins, dentures, wires, battery, etc.
- Radiolucent FB's are plastic toys, beads, wooden objects, etc.

SITES

Most common site of lodgment is at the physiologic or pathologic narrowings.

Physiological Narrowings

- Cricopharyngeal sphincter—present at C6 vertebral level and 15 cm from upper incisors
- Crossing of arch of aorta—at T4 vertebral level and 25 cm from upper incisors
- Crossing of left bronchus—at T5 vertebral level and 27 cm from upper incisors
- Right crus of diaphragm—at T10 vertebral level and 40 cm from upper incisors.

Pathological Narrowings

- Benign and malignant strictures
- Malignant growths
- Scar from burn and surgery
- Scleroderma
- Diffuse esophageal spasm or achalasia.

Pathological Changes Caused by the FB

- Button, batteries and sharp FB, such as safety pin, may rapidly lead to complications like esophageal perforation, severe inflammation with resultant strictures and tracheoesophageal fistula[3]
- Coins may stay in the esophagus for many months and cause only a slow ulceration of esophageal wall
- Meat and fish bone will very soon give rise to ulceration, periesophagitis and other complications like mediastinitis and deep space neck infection.[1] History of fish bone impaction is usually of recent onset but sometimes patient may present with old retained foreign body with complications. Sometimes, small fish bone in the lower pole of tonsil adjoining to the base of tongue may enter tongue and is propagated anteriorly into the body of the tongue by muscular contractions[4]
- Migration of FB—rarely FB penetrates the wall of aerodigestive tract and even more rarely they do migrate in soft tissue and viscera of neck. The sharper the FB the higher the risk of penetration. The risk of penetration is also influenced by the FB's orientation; horizontally oriented FB is likely to penetrate. Perforating and migrating. FB can introduce bacteria into the soft tissue of the neck and cause suppurative complications such as para or retropharyngeal abscess. Infection can spread into the mediastinum and lead to life-threatening mediastinitis. FB might also penetrate adjacent visceral structures such as thyroid gland, the major blood vessels in the neck and precipitate vascular complications such as aortoesophageal and innominate esophageal and carotid rupture.[5]

Ching Ping Wang[6] (2009) reported a migrating fish bone presenting as acute onset of neck lump. CT scan showed diffuse emphysema over the subcutaneous and deep layers of neck and the needle-like radiopaque density that penetrated the left sternomastoid muscle at the level of thyroid cartilage. In this case, perforation of upper aerodigestive tract was present due to migrating foreign body.

Jiannis Hajiioannou MD et al.[7] (2011) reported migration of an impacted pharyngeal foreign body of the hypopharynx to the prevertebral space, after an unsuccessful attempt of endoscopic removal.

CLINICAL FEATURES

Symptomatology

- Pain
    - Adult patient: History of foreign body ingestion is usually elicited. Patient may be able to give a very accurate account of the type and shape of FB swallowed
        - He is very often able to point to the exact site of the obstruction, particularly if the FB is lodging in the upper third of esophagus
        - When FB is in the middle or lower third of the esophagus, localization is not so accurate and pain is referred to the back or behind the sternum. Pain is of a sharp, cutting nature, is worse with attempts to swallow and occurs at the same place every time the patient swallows
        - A smooth FB may give rise to only a vague sensation of discomfort and not to actual pain
        - Vague discomfort in the epigastrium suggests that the FB is entrapped at the lower esophageal sphincter
    - Children: Children who cannot give history, the presence of a particularly smooth FB may be unsuspected for several months. The history is given by a parent, who has seen the child with an object in his or her mouth and suspects the child might have swallowed it. Gagging, vomiting, neck or throat pain or refusal to swallow may give indication of foreign body ingestion in these patients
- Dysphagia is nearly always present, and is due to the size of FB or inflammatory reaction and spasm caused by its presence. Initially, only slight difficulty in swallowing may be present, but later the difficulty becomes more pronounced
- Regurgitation of food and later regurgitation of blood-stained saliva and mucus is present[1]
- Difficulty in breathing: Since, the party wall between the trachea and esophagus is thin and deformable, esophageal FB often present with respiratory distress, in addition to drooling and dysphagia.[3]

Evaluation (Examination) of Patient

After thorough history, patient must be observed during the act of swallowing. When sharp FB is lodged in the upper part of esophagus, its introitus (pyriform fossa and post-cricoid region) or in the larynx, swallowing gives a definite expression of pain. The oropharynx is well-innervated and patient can typically localize oropharyngeal foreign body. Scratches or abrasions to the mucosal surface of the oropharynx can create FB sensation.

Neck Examination

Examination of neck may show a tender swelling in the lower part of neck medial to sternomastoid muscle; this swelling is usually caused by:

- The inflammatory reaction around the FB
- Actual abscess
- Surgical emphysema, which is recognized by accompanied crepitus.

Tenderness—on pressure, on the trachea may be present. This is considered pathognomonic of the presence of a FB in the cervical esophagus. On movement of the trachea and larynx towards the point of maximum tenderness, there is marked exacerbation of pain.

Oropharyngeal examination—Fish bone or sharp foreign body may be visible in oropharynx. Lower pole of tonsil, particularly near its attachment with tongue should be particularly looked for, in case of small sharp FB, e.g. Fish bone, wire, etc. Indirect laryngoscopy should be done for lodgment of FB in base of tongue, vallecula and superficial part of pyriform fossa. Drooling of saliva suggests obstruction in pyriform fossa, post-cricoid region or cricopharynx.

Each part of pharyngeal wall must be minutely studied in the mirror; otherwise, the tip of small fish bone almost completely buried in the tissue will be overlooked. If the patient can localize his pain to one side or other, then the FB or the laceration caused by its passage must be above the cricoid level and should be visible in the mirror.

If no FB can be seen in the laryngeal mirror, further investigations are necessary.

Radiological Examination

Plain films of neck and chest are taken. Ideally, both the anteroposterior and lateral views are taken to know the exact location and disposition of the FB.

Foreign body (FB) in the esophagus, particularly flat objects like coins lie in the coronal plane in contrast to laryngeal or tracheal FB, which lies in the sagittal plane (Figures 8.1 to 8.4). It is very important to repeat X-rays prior to general anesthesia, if more than 2 hours have passed since the original film.

If the FB is not revealed, the neck, thorax and abdomen are screened. If an opaque shadow is still not seen, a little barium sulfate is given and its passage down

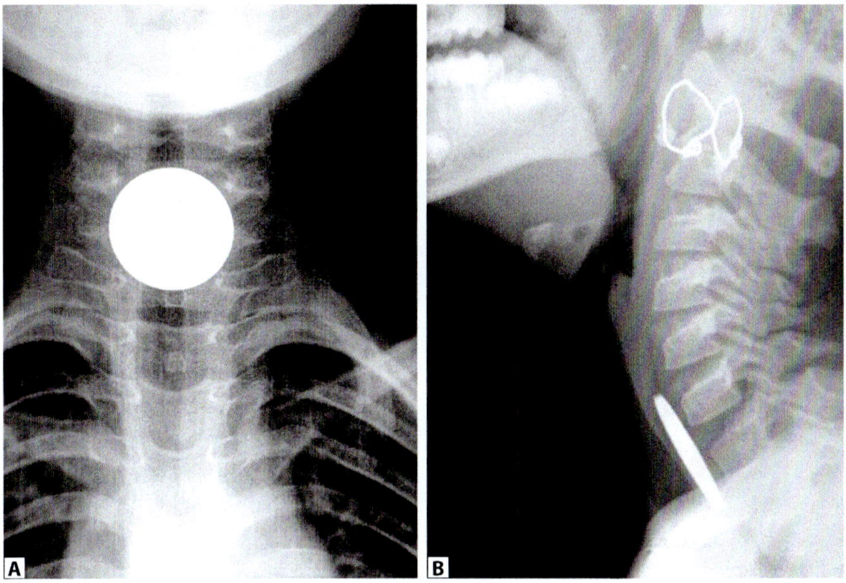

Figures 8.1A and B Plain X-ray of skull, neck and upper thorax (anteroposterior and lateral views) showing round metallic FB (coin) in upper esophagus (C6 to T1)

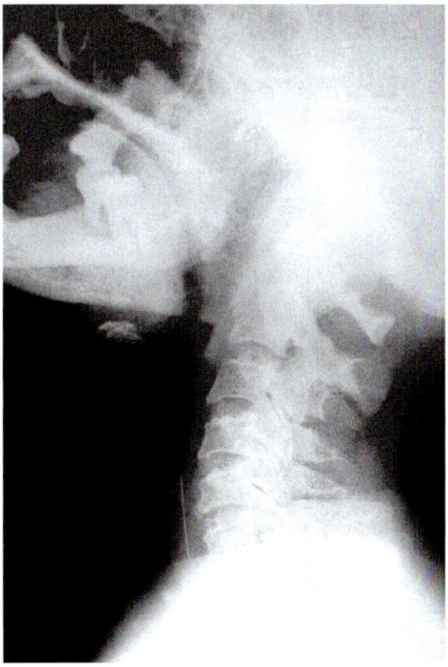

Figure 8.2 Plain X-ray of skull, neck and upper thorax (lateral view) showing a fish bone in pyriform fossa and cervical esophagus (C6 to C7)

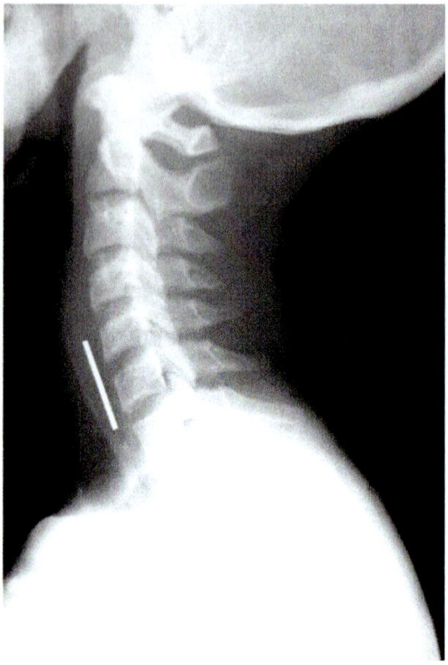

Figure 8.3 Plain X-ray of skull, neck and upper thorax (lateral view) showing a safety pin in cervical esophagus (C6 to C7)

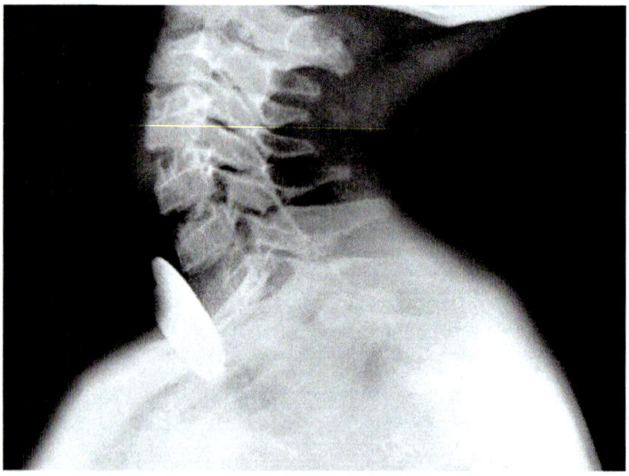

Figure 8.4 Plain X-ray of skull, neck and upper thorax (lateral view) showing an almost round metallic FB in upper esophagus (C7 to T2)

the gullet is observed. The opaque medium may be held up at one point and may actually outline the FB or the flow of barium may be split. If the barium cannot be easily dislodged by further swallowing or washed down with water, the presence of FB is to be strongly suspected. An air bubble in the esophagus, in the region of the hold-up, is very often indicative of FB.

Another technique for visualizing non-opaque FB is to have patient swallow small piece of cotton impregnated with barium paste. The cotton wool will become lodged with the non-opaque FB and will reveal its presence and position.[1] Barium is contraindicated in cases, in which esophageal perforation is suspected.

While evaluating the lateral neck radiograph for FB in hypopharynx and cervical esophagus, some radiodensities may be misinterpreted as being caused by FB.

- Partial calcification of the posterior aspect of the thyroid or cricoid cartilages is often misinterpreted as an FB in the cervical esophagus
- The thyroid ligament (cartilago triticea) may be calcified
- The superior and inferior horns of the thyroid cartilage often project posteriorly and may be misinterpreted as FB
- The stylohyoid ligament may be calcified
- The ear lobe may cast shadow on the hypopharynx or pharynx
- Calcium deposits in the carotid artery, salivary glands, lymph nodes or thyroid adenoma may also be interpreted as FB.[8]

CT scan: If the FB is small and nonopaque, diagnosis is difficult and CT scan is indicated. It should also be done in cases of suspected perforation or abscess.

Management

Most foreign bodies, which can be seen with the mirror, can be removed without recourse to general anesthesia.

Removal of FB with the help of mirror examination:

- Explain the procedure to the patient
- Heat the laryngeal mirror; confirm that it is not too hot
- Ask the patient to hold his tongue in a gauge piece
- Surgeon holds the mirror in his left hand and a pair of suitably-angled grasping forceps in his right hand
- With the help of mirror, the forceps is guided down the throat until the FB can be grasped and removed. Care must be taken that, there must of course be no blind 'grab'
- Every step must be clearly observed in the mirror.

There is no greater reward in laryngology than to see the relief and gratitude of a patient, who in a matter of moments, is relieved of a fish bone in the pharynx. This technique, which requires a little practice, is well worth cultivating.[1]

If no FB can be seen in the laryngeal mirror, further investigations and endoscopy is imperative. Nasal endoscopy or fiberoptic nasopharyngoscopy can be done in these cases. Even if the symptoms improve rapidly, the patient must be kept under observation until he is completely symptom free. Abrasion of the esophageal mucosa will give some pain and cause dysphagia, but usually these symptoms disappear rapidly.

Increase of pain and dysphagia indicates the presence of a FB or some more serious damage to the esophageal wall and warrants more active treatment, such as endoscopic examination.[2]

Treatment

Although esophagoscopy for the removal of FB may be an emergency operation, the surgeon must have knowledge of the nature, size and site of the foreign body and, if possible, a replica should be examined.

Coin in the Esophagus of a Child

The radiological examination must be repeated immediately before the endoscopy is done, because the coin may have passed into the stomach, if there has been a delay between first seeing the patient and endoscopic examination. Small negus type (35 cm in length) esophagoscope, esophageal speculum, or even an anterior commissure laryngoscope can be used. In case of FB impacted in upper end of esophagus, the instrument should be passed slowly, because it is very easy to override the foreign body, especially if it has been in the esophagus where it is coated with mucus. Any food debris is removed by suction. Esophagoscope is passed as near to the foreign body as possible, making sure not to push the foreign body ahead. Coin should be maintained in the center of the field. Alligator forceps is then passed and the coin is seized firmly and brought out until it impinges on the end of esophagoscope. The forceps is fixed by the surgeon at the proximal end of the esophagoscope so that the FB, forceps and esophagoscope can be pulled out of the esophagus together. Care must be taken when the FB is passing the cricopharyngeus, that the coin is turned so that it lies in the coronal plane. Otherwise, it may slip off and may be found lying in the hypopharynx; for its removal, a laryngoscope is then necessary.

A Sharp Foreign Body in the Esophagus

A sharp FB may be a meat bone or a fish bone, which may get lodged anywhere in the esophagus, and the anesthetist must take care not to pass endotracheal tube blindly because it may accidentally go into the esophagus and cause the FB to perforate the esophageal wall. The surgeon must resist any temptation to extract the FB without noting the position of its sharp edge.

Mucus, food debris and any barium, which has been left after an X-ray examination, are removed by suction. If the ends of the FB are free, the forceps is passed and the end is gripped. If any bleeding occurs a swab soaked in adrenaline is introduced. If the ends of the FB are buried in the esophageal wall, manipulation is necessary to try to release one end and to get a point of the FB into the tube so that its long axis is parallel to the esophagoscope.

A small bone may be extracted through the esophagoscope, but a large one should be rated as for a coin and removed with esophagoscope and forceps. Patient must be kept under close observation because this type of the FB is likely to cause complications.

Meat and Soft Foreign Bodies

Meat and soft foreign bodies are extracted piece meal. Cancer of the esophagus may present as a case of an impacted food bolus. Therefore, after endoscopic removal of the impacted meat or other food, it is important to pass the esophagoscope again and to check that there is no underlying intrinsic esophageal lesion.

Safety-pin in the Esophagus

An open safety-pin presents no difficulty, if the sharp point is distal. If the point is proximal there is often great difficulty and, several methods have been devised to overcome it. If it is not too large it may be possible to turn the pin in the esophagus, or alternatively to manipulate the point of the pin into the lumen of the esophagus. Some endoscopists prefer to cut the pin in situ using endoscopic shears, or to close it with Clerf's or similar forceps. If all else fails, the pin may be grasped with rotation forceps at the ring, pushed into the stomach and allowed to rotate and then be extracted through the esophagus with the point trailing.

Denture in the Esophagus

A denture in the esophagus presents many hazards. The radiograph should be studied carefully with special regard to the hooks and points on the denture. During esophagoscopy, the hook should, if possible, be manipulated into the lumen of the esophagus before extraction. The denture may be impacted and may have to be divided in situ. If there is gross trauma of the esophagus by the foreign body or if any previous manipulation has been performed, endoscopic removal should be delayed, and it is better to wait until the inflammatory reaction has subsided and do the esophagoscopy some days later. In the meantime, the patient should be treated as for a periesophagitis or perforation of the esophagus with systemic antibiotics.[1]

On removing FB, there is sometimes an obvious underlying lesion such as benign or malignant stricture. These should be biopsied and appropriate investigation instituted. On removing the endoscope, a careful check should be made for mucosal tear that may have occurred during extraction. In case of doubt about this, a nasogastric tube should be carefully passed and patient should be kept nil by mouth until a chest radiograph has been performed and patient is observed for 24 hours. If there is history of recurrent impaction, videofluoroscopy should be performed to rule out motility disorder or a psychiatric assessment arranged if appropriate. Jone, Lannigan and Salma (1991) advocated a follow-up barium swallow in all patients with bolus obstruction.

Battery Ingestion

Button batteries may appear as coin-shaped objects on radiographs, but should be treated as surgical emergency. It causes tissue destruction rapidly and can culminate in an esophageal perforation after several hours. Battery can cause direct pressure and low voltage electrical burns leading to tissue injury. The removal of battery is difficult because of the associated inflammation and its slippery nature. Battery can be pushed into the stomach, as there is usually little damage to the lower gastrointestinal tract. If the battery cannot be retrieved or manipulated in to the stomach then open removal may be necessary. Following removal of the battery from the esophagus, follow-up radiology should be arranged at intervals to exclude the late development of stricture.

Medical Treatment

Pharmacological agents such as glucagons have been used successfully in promoting the passage of meat boluses since first described by Ferrucci and Long (1977). The method is thought to work by reducing lower esophageal sphincter pressure (Smith, 1986). The technique works in around 40% of patients presumably because it does not affect the diameter of strictures or rings. A 1 to 2 mg IV bolus may cause nausea, vomiting or hyperglycemia, but it is usually well-tolerated. Historical attempts to digest meat boluses enzymatically with proteolytic agents such as papain, have now fallen from favor, because of two potentially life-threatening complications of enzymes—transmural digestion (Holsinger, Fuson and Sealy, 1968) of the esophagus and hemorrhagic pulmonary edema, if the compound is aspirated. In addition, alternative conservative measure is to use agents, which release gas into the esophagus, thus raising intraluminal pressure, distending the esophagus against the closed cricopharyngeal muscle and thus, interiorly forcing the bolus into the stomach. The gas forming agents include simple carbonated drinks, a cocktail of tartaric acid and sodium bicarbonate and Carbex effervescent granules (sodium bicarbonate, activated dimethicone and citric acid).

Flexible Endoscopy

At some of the center, the flexible fiberoptic endoscopy is preferred, but it lacks the advantages of rigid endoscopy. Flexible endoscopy does, however, offer the advantage of allowing examination of the stomach and duodenum in the event of no FB being found in esophagus. Flexible endoscopy may be used when rigid endoscopy is contraindicated.[2]

Advantages of Rigid Endoscopy

- It provides the benefit of protected airway
- It limits the risk of converting an esophageal FB to laryngotracheal FB, during extraction

- Optical forceps can be used with it, giving excellent visualization and firm control of the object.

External Operation for Removal of FB

The following types of foreign bodies may require removal by the external route:

- An impacted FB
- A foreign body producing periesophagitis after unsuccessful attempts at removal through the esophagoscope
- A periesophageal abscess with foreign body lodging in the abscess itself.

Complications of FB

- Respiratory obstruction: This is due to tracheal compression by FB in esophagus or laryngeal edema, especially in infants and children
- Periesophageal cellulitis and abscess in neck
- Perforation: Sharp objects may perforate the esophageal wall, setting up mediastinitis, pericarditis or empyema. They may perforate the aorta and prove fatal
- Rarely tracheoesophageal fistula
- Ulceration and Stricture: Over looked FB may cause slow ulceration and stricture.[1]

Caustic Ingestion

It occurs most commonly in children or suicidal adults. In children, the volume ingested is small, as they are deterred by the foul taste of most toxic substances, but it could be higher in adults with intentional ingestion.

Evaluation of Patient

History and identification of ingested substance should be sought. Alkali (pH>7) ingestion leads to liquefaction necrosis with deep esophageal injuries. Acidic (pH<7) substance, e.g. battery fluid cause corrosive injury, which frequently is limited to mucosa. Household bleach usually has pH around 7, it may irritate esophageal mucosa and, permanent sequelae are uncommon.

Careful evaluation of entire upper aerodigestive tract should be done. Oral and pharyngeal injuries are common, especially with acid ingestion (foul tasting acidic substances stimulates gagging and retching). Water or milk ingestion dilutes the substance and there may be some benefit from this in some patients. Gastric lavage and emetics are strictly contraindicated in caustic ingestion.

Role of Endoscopy

- If ingested substance is believed to be injurious or unknown.

- Best performed between 24 to 48 hours after injury. The amount of damage may be underestimated, if endoscopy is performed too early (<12 hours) and further delay increases the risk of perforation during endoscopy. Esophagography may be considered. In case of suspected perforation, flexible esophagoscopy is contraindicated.

Grading of Injury

According to extent of mucosal injury:
Grade1: Superficial injuries (do not usually lead to permanent sequelae and do not usually require treatment).
Grade 2: Transmucosal injury (high risk of stricture formation).
Grade 3: Transmural injury (high risk for perforation and stricture and almost always require surgical intervention).

Circumferential injuries are more likely to lead to late complications. If possible nasogastric tube should be passed during endoscopy in grade 2 and grade 3.
Role of steroid: Controversial and should be avoided.
Role of antibiotics: Given in perforation and secondary infection.
Role of antireflux therapy: May be of some benefit in preventing strictures.

LATE COMPLICATIONS

- Stricture formation (needing serial endoscopic dilatation or resection)
- Risk of developing carcinoma. Patient should be kept under regular follow-up.[3]

REFERENCES

1. Scott-Brown's Diseases of the Ear, Nose and Throat, 4th edition. 1979;4:237-43.
2. Scott-Brown's Otolaryngology, 6th edition. page 5/1/11 and 5/24/22.
3. Ballenger's Otolaryngology and Head and Neck Surgery, 17th edition. 2008;980-1.
4. Saha S, Chandra S, et al. Emergency Otorhinolaryngological cases in Medical College Kolkata: a statistical analysis. Ind J Otolaryngol Head and Neck Surgery. 2005;57(3): 219-25.
5. Al-Sebeih K, Valvoda M, et al. Perforating and migrating pharyngoesophageal foreign bodies. ENT-Ear, Nose and Throat (Kuwait). 2006;85(9):600-3.
6. Wang CP, Jiang SL. Migrating fish bone presenting as acute onset of neck lump. Formus Medical Association. 2009;108(2):170-2.
7. Hajiioannou J, et al. Otorhinolaryngologia–Head and Neck Surgery. 2011;43:30-4.
8. Montgomery WW. Surgery of the Larynx, Trachea, Esophagus and Neck. 2002.p. 23, 30.

CHAPTER

9 Emergency in Maxillofacial Injuries

Synonyms: *Facial trauma, facial fractures, upper and lower jaw fractures or broken jaws.*

INTRODUCTION

Maxillofacial trauma or injuries (Figures 9.1 and 9.2) are commonly encountered in the practice of emergency medicine and are presenting one of the most challenging problems to the attending surgeons or physicians in the emergency outpatient's department. Fractures of the facial skeleton are associated with variable morbidity, disfigurement and functional deficits. More than 50% of these patients have multisystem trauma requiring coordinated management between

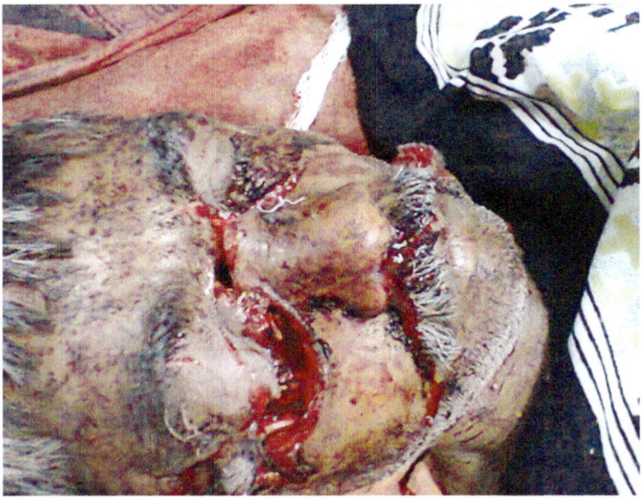

Figure 9.1 LeFort III fracture

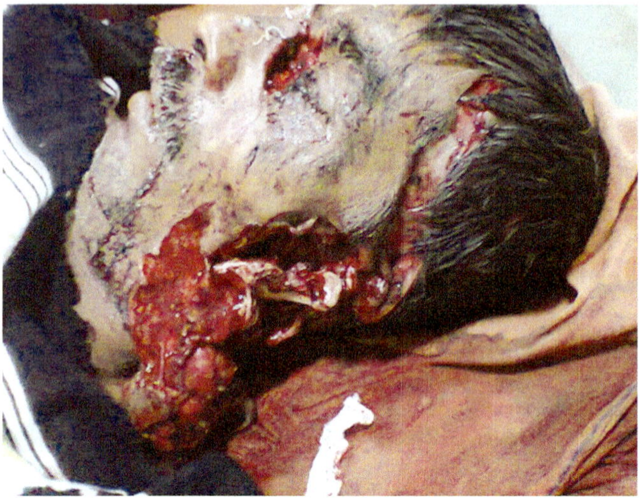

Figure 9.2 Maxillofacial trauma

physician, otorhinolaryngologist, trauma surgeon, ophthalmologist, dentist, oral and faciomaxillary surgeon and neurosurgeons altogether. Maxillofacial trauma includes injuries to any of the bony or fleshy structures of the face. A fractured nose or jaw may affect the ability to breathe or eat. Any maxillofacial injury may also prevent the passage of air or be severe enough to cause a concussion or more serious brain damage.

Road traffic accidents are reported to be the most common causes in developing countries whereas interpersonal violence is the leading cause in the developed countries.[1] With regards to the anatomical sites, mandibular and zygomatic complex fractures account for the majorities among all types of facial fracture.[2] Males are more predominant sufferer than females. Their occurrence varies according to the mechanism of injury and demographic factors like sex, age, race, geographic distribution, culture, socioeconomic status and road safety regulations.[2] The trauma to this region is very much concerned with function of the various special organs like eyes, ear, nose, mouth, and vital structures of head and neck. Also, the psychological impact of disfigurement after the injuries can be devastating.

ANATOMICAL CONSIDERATIONS

The maxillofacial region is divided into three different parts (Figures 9.3 and 9.4).

- Upper face: This includes frontal bone and sinus
- Midface: The midface contains the nasal bones, ethmoid, zygoma and maxilla. This is divided into upper and lower parts.
- Upper part

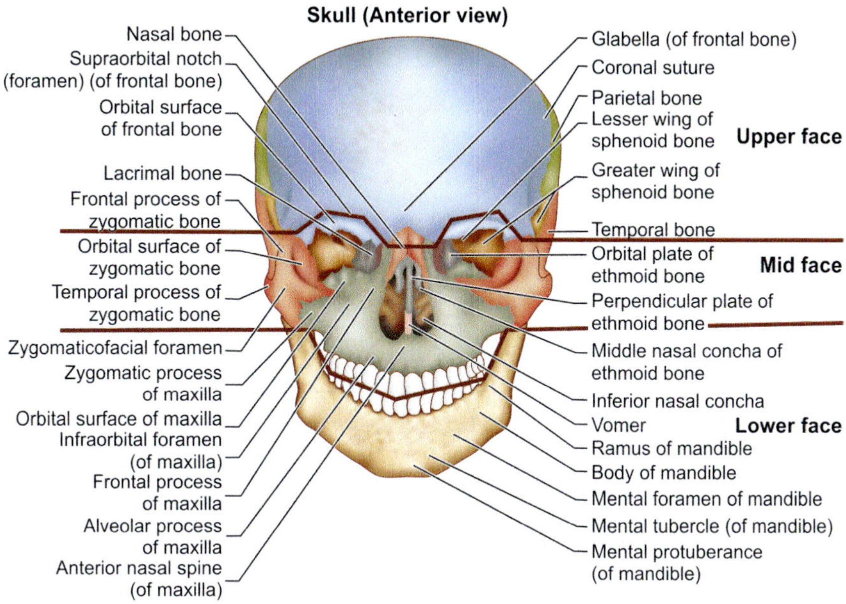

Figure 9.3 Frontal view of the skull

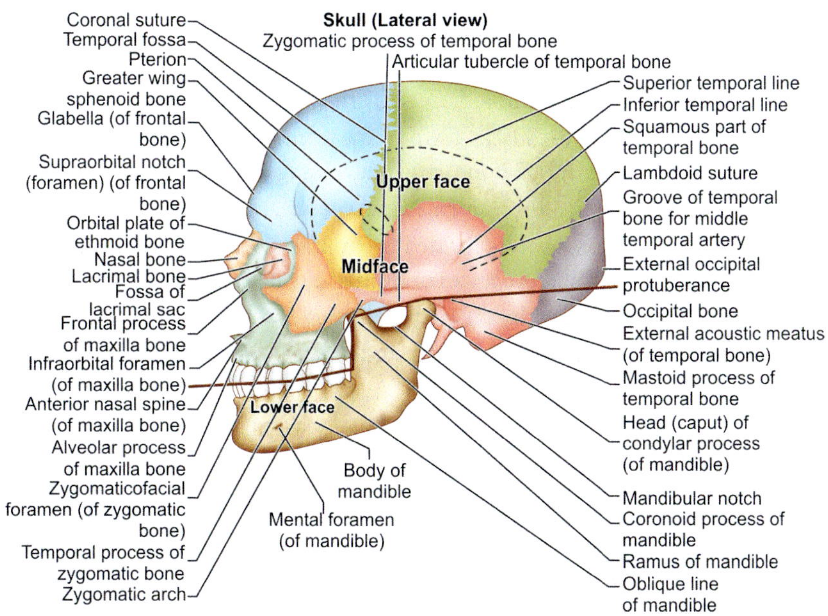

Figure 9.4 Lateral view of the skull with subdivisions

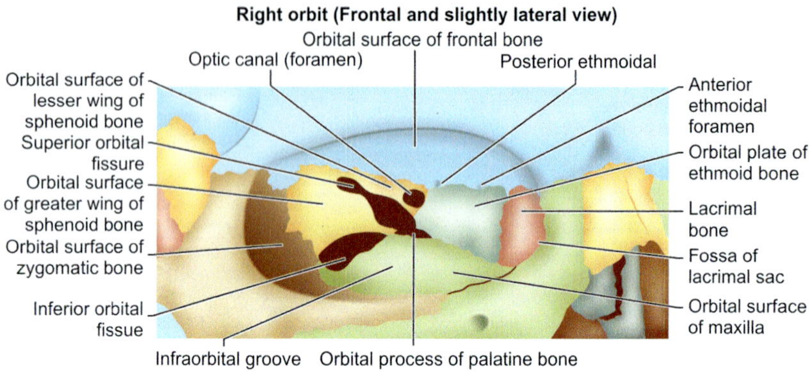

Figure 9.5 The orbit

- That part of maxilla where LeFort II and LeFort III fractures occur
- Nose, nasoethmoid complex, zygomaticomaxillary complex and orbit

- Lower part
  - Where LeFort I fracture occurs
- Lower face: This part includes the mandible having its condyle, ramus, angle, body, symphysis, alveolar part and coronoid process.

The Orbit

The orbit needs separate description because of its complexity in formation. The parts of the orbit are (Figure 9.5):

- Superior orbital margin—this is formed by the frontal bone
- Lateral orbital margin—this is formed by frontal process of zygoma, the zygomatic process of frontal bone and greater wing of sphenoid
- Inferior orbital margin—this is formed by zygoma and maxilla
- Medial orbital margin—this is formed by frontal process of maxilla, lacrimal bone, angular and orbital processes of frontal and ethmoid bones
- The orbital floor is formed by the roof of maxilla
- The apex—this is formed by the lesser and greater wing of sphenoid, palatine and part of ethmoid.

THE NERVES

The maxillofacial area is innervated or related by all cranial nerves, but major innervations are from the trigeminal nerve, facial nerve and great auricular nerve through the branches.

Trigeminal Nerve

- Ophthalmic division—first division of trigeminal nerve
  - Sensory supply—to the skin of forehead, upper lid and conjunctiva
  - Branches
    - Lacrimal nerve
    - Supraorbital nerve
    - Supratrochlear nerve
    - External laryngeal nerve
    - Nasocilliary nerve
    - Frontal nerve
- Maxillary division—second division of trigeminal nerve
  - Sensory supply—to the skin of part of nose, lower eyelid, cheek and upper lip
  - Branches
    - Infraorbital nerve
    - Zygomaticofacial nerve
    - Zgomaticotemporal nerve
    - Anterior and posterior alveolar nerve
- Mandibular division—third division of trigeminal nerve
  - Motor supply to the muscles of mastication
  - Sensory supply—to the skin of lower lip, chin, temporal area, and part of auricle
  - Branches
    - Lingual nerve
    - Inferior alveolar nerve
    - Zygomaticofacial nerve
    - Dental nerve
    - Mental nerve
    - Buccal nerve
    - Auriculotemporal nerve.

Facial Nerve

The facial nerve supplies motor innervations to all muscles of facial expression through the branches like:

- Zygomaticofacial
- Faciocervical branches.

Greater Auricular Nerve

This is a branch of cervical plexus that supplies the angle of the mandible, and skin over the parotid and mastoid process.

Other Cranial Nerves

- CN-I (Olfactory nerve)—for smell
- CN-II (Optic nerve)—for vision
- CN-III (Occulomotor nerve)—for eyeball movement with superior, medial and inferior recti, inferior oblique, levator palpebrae, pupilloconstrictor and ciliary muscles
- CN-IV (Trochlear nerve)—eyeball movement through innervation of superior oblique
- CN-VI (Abducens nerve)—eyeball movement through innervation of lateral rectus
- CN-VIII (Vestibulocohlear nerve)—for hearing and balance
- CN-IX (Glossopharyngeal nerve)—for taste, swallowing and salivation
- CN-X (Vagus nerve)—for taste, swallowing and palate elevation
- CN-XI (Spinal accessory nerve)—head rotation and shrugging
- CN-XII (Hypoglossal nerve)—movement of tongue.

BLOOD SUPPLY

The face is highly vascular area of the body and is mainly supplied by branches of external carotid artery through the lingual, facial, internal maxillary and superficial temporal arteries and venous drainage is through superficial temporal, pterygoid, retromandibular, lingual, facial, and external jugular veins.

INCIDENCE AND PREVALENCE

Information regarding the demographic distribution of the maxillofacial injuries depends very often upon various factors like country, location of trauma center, reporting facilities available, urban or rural age groups, sex and overall influence implication of rule and regulation of the land in respect of traffic, Labor Acts and child abuse, etc. on its population. Universally, many literatures show that the most active period of life, i.e. second to third decade of life is the commonest age group to be affected by maxillofacial injuries.[4,7,8] Youth are frequently involved in high speed transportation, outdoor contact sports and engage acts of affray.[8] In a study ZA Rana et al., (2010) pointed out that about 73% patients were males, signifying the male gender predominance, which is also consistent with literatures from around the world.[4-6] Falls account for 78% of facial injuries in preschoolers and 47% of such injuries in children between the ages of 6 and 15. In older adolescents and adults, violent crime or other personal assaults account for almost 50% of facial injuries, with automobile accidents accounting for 29% and sports-related accidents for another 11%. Patients between the ages of 17 and 30 are more likely to suffer facial injuries from gunshot wounds, while older adults are more likely to be injured by attacks with blunt objects. About 10% of facial injuries in young children are caused by parental abuse. Children who grow up on farms are at significant risk for injury by animals.[3]

ETIOLOGY

In a study ZA Rana et al., (2010) demonstrated that road traffic accidents account maximum (57%) followed by fall (11%), and natural disaster (10%).[4] In urban setup community, causes of faciomaxillary trauma are mostly due to assaults, road traffic accidents, zygomatic and mandible are most commonly encountered fractures due to assaults. In community and rural setup population, motor vehicle accidents, assaults, recreational activities, accidents are the main causes for faciomaxillary trauma. Other causes of faciomaxillary trauma include falls from the height, sports injury, gunshots, fire arm injury, occupational, penetrating trauma, domestic violence, child abuse and natural calamities. Some other studies as reported by Bataineh AB from Jordan (55%), Subhasraj et al., from India (62%), Laski R et al., from USA (40%), Schatenaar K et al., from England (24.7%), Cheema F, from Pakistan (44%), and Leles JL Rodrigues et al., from Brazil (45.7%) also significantly denote that the road traffic accident is the single most common etiological factor for causing the maxillofacial injuries.[7,9-13] In pediatric age group, the causes of facial trauma include falls (most common), blunt trauma, by sports activities, motor vehicles accidents, assaults, non-accidental trauma, and child abuse. In children maxillofacial trauma is associated with soft tissue injury (most common), injury to cervical spine and, intracranial injury.[3] Okoje, Alonge, Oluteye et al. in their study on changing pattern of pediatric maxillofacial injuries in Ibadan, Nigeria demonstrated that the RTA scored highest among all etiological factors (54.5%) followed by falls (35.8%) from height causing maxillofacial injuries.[14]

PATHOPHYSIOLOGY

The kinetic energy present in a moving object is a function of the mass multiplied by the square of its velocity. The dispersion of the kinetic energy during deceleration produces the force that results in injury. High impact and low impact forces are defined as greater or lesser than the 50 times the force of gravity. The supraorbital rim, symphysis and condyle and angle of mandible and frontal bones require a high impact force to be damaged and zygoma, and nasal bones require low impact force to be damaged (Table 9.1).[15]

Contradictory to the adults, because of the differences in the proportion of a child's head and skeleton, relative prominence of child's cranium compared to the midface, together with the elasticity of the immature facial skeleton, the incidence of fractures of facial skeleton in children is very low. In comparison, a child suffers more soft tissue injury than maxillofacial trauma in the form of laceration, burn

Table 9.1 Force required for facial bone fractures[28]

Bone	*Force of gravity (g)*
Nasal bones	30
Zygomatic bones	50
Angle of mandible bones	70
Frontal glabellar region bones	80
Midline maxilla bones	100
Midline mandible bones	100
Supraorbital bones	200

and electrical trauma. Considering the clinical aspects of maxillofacial trauma, the high incidence of nasal and zygomatico-orbital complex fractures is obviously related to the prominent position of these structures within facial skeleton and their proximity to the external trauma.[16,17] Road traffic accidents are the main cause of dentoalveolar fractures especially in motorbike accidents where security measures are neglected.[18]

As far as mandible is concerned, the most common site of mandibular fractures due to assaults is the mandible angle[19,20] and greater incidence of condyle fracture is observed in traffic accidents.[21] The age associated risks of injuries resulting from falls differ in two ways. In children, it is due to incomplete motor development and greater craniofacial mass to body ratio that leads to greater incidence of maxillofacial injury.[25,26] Whereas in elderly it is due to neuromuscular and motor limitations that leads to greater incidence of maxillofacial injury.[20,27]

DIFFERENT FRACTURES

Upper Face

- *Frontal bone and sinus fractures:* In frontal bone fractures, which require severe blow to the forehead, the anterior and posterior tables may be fractured and sometimes the dura may be tore in posterior table fractures and nasofrontal duct is injured in anterior table fracture.[22] Fractures of frontal bone may occur in association with extensive facial injuries as a result of direct blunt trauma to the forehead in motor vehicle accidents, sporting collision or assaults
- *Nasal bone fractures:* Nasal bone fractures result in forces transmitted during trauma. Isolated nasal bone fractures are the most commonly seen fractures in facial trauma but this may be associated with severe midface trauma involving naso-orbito-ethmoidal complex the frontal sinus and orbito-zygomatic complex. Nasal and zygomatico-orbital fractures are mostly due to RTA (road traffic accidents), and assaults.[23,24]

Midface

Upper Central

- *Orbital floor fractures:* The orbital floor fracture can occur in isolation or in association with medial wall fracture. When a force strikes the globe or orbital rim, the intraorbital pressure increases with transmission of this force and damages the weakest aspect of the orbit, i.e. the floor and medial wall. Herniation of the orbital contents into the maxillary sinus is possible. The incidence of ocular injury is high but globe rupture is rare
- *Nasoethmoid complex fractures:* The fracture extends from the nose to the ethmoid and can result in damage to medial canthus, lacrimal apparatus, nasofrontal duct, dura and cribriform plate.

Lateral Midface

- *Zygomatic arch fracture:* This is caused by direct blow and can result in isolated fracture of zygomaticotemporal suture. The arch tends to break at its weakest point, which lies just posterior to the zygomaticotemporal suture line. A direct blow may cause fracture of the orbital floor producing a blowout. The displacement is usually to the medial direction and can produce trismus by interfering with coronoid process and temporalis muscles. If the temporalis and masseteric fascia are disrupted the arch tends to collapse inferiorly.
- Zygomaticomaxillary complex fracture: Zygomaticomaxillary complex fractures resulting from the direct trauma extend through zygomaticofrontal and zygomaticomaxillary sutures. The fracture lines usually extend through the infraorbital foramen and orbital floor. Ocular injury is common. These fractures are also known as tripod fractures. Two factors usually govern the degree and type of displacement of bone. First, the direction and site of the impact relative to the axis of the zygomatic bone and the second, the pull of the masseter and the integrity of the fascial attachments.

Lower Central Midface

Maxillary Fractures

These fractures are traditionally divided into alveolar, LeFort I, II, III fractures as most of them follow the lines of weakness.

- Alveolar: This can occur in isolation from a direct low energy force through the alveolar line
- LeFort I (Guerin) fracture or horizontal or transmaxillary fracture (Figures 9.6A and B): Here is a horizontal maxillary fracture that runs across the inferior aspect of maxilla and separates alveolar process and hard palate from the rest

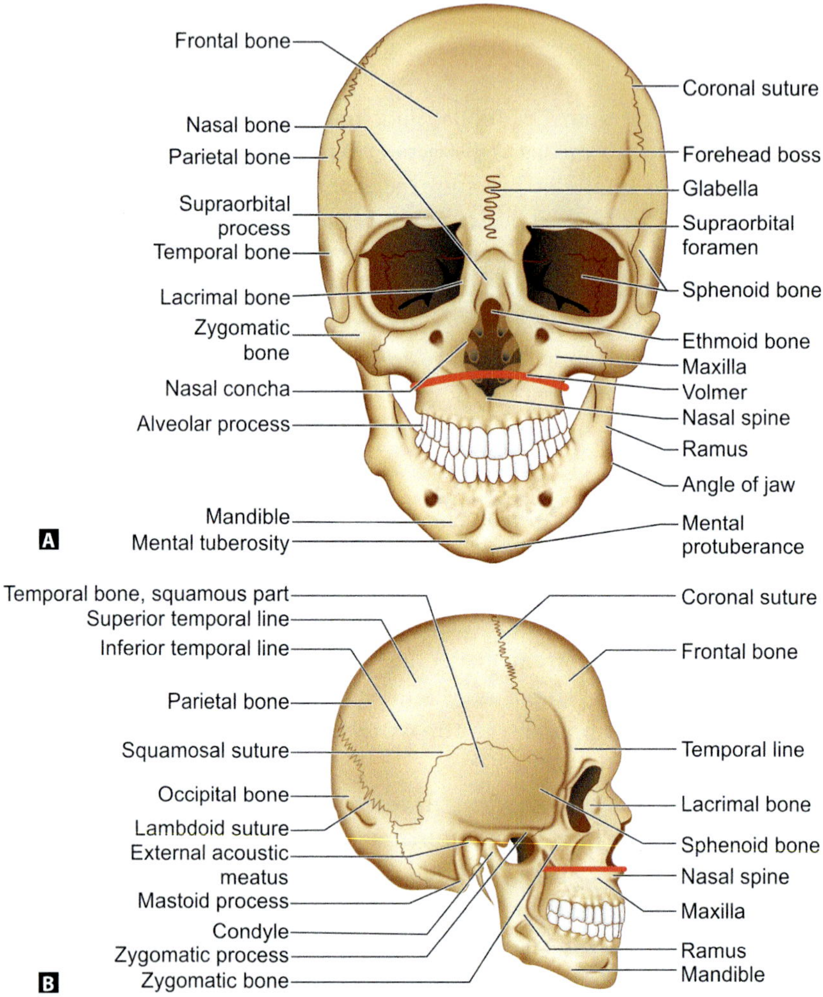

Figures 9.6A and B LeFort I (Guerin) fracture. (A) Frontal view; (B) Lateral view

of the maxilla. This extends through the lower third of nasal septum, maxillary sinuses, inferior part of medial and lateral pterygoid plates, and palatine bones resulting in a mobile maxilla with a stable upper midface. This complicates with loss of teeth infection and malocclusion

- *LeFort II (pyramidal) fracture (Figures 9.7A and B):* Due to its triangular shape, this is called a pyramidal fracture. This type of fracture involves separation through frontal process, lacrimal bone, floor of orbit zygomaticomaxillary suture line, lateral wall of maxillary sinuses, pterygoid plates. Maxilla and nose are mobile. This fracture involves the non-union of fractured bones, obstruction to the tear duct and lacrimal gland, double vision and malocclusion

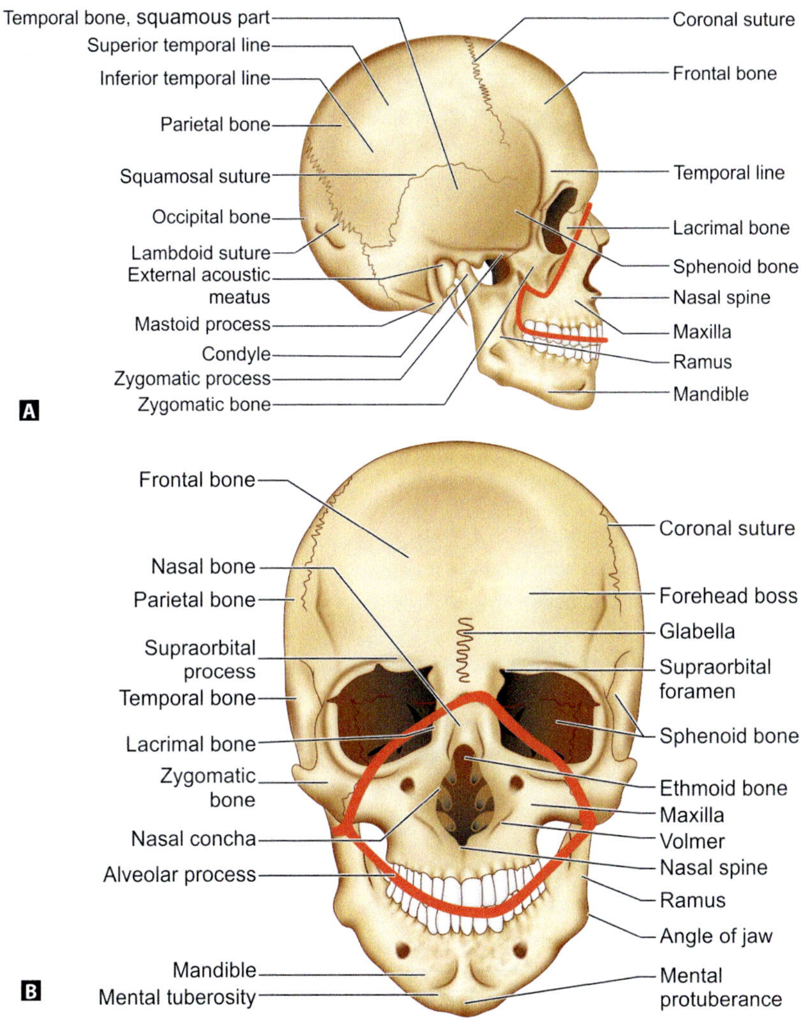

Figures 9.7A and B LeFort II (pyramidal) fracture. (A) Lateral view; (B) Frontal view

- *LeFort III or craniofacial disjunction or dislocation (Figures 9.8A and B):* This is a very severe kind of fracture and may be associated with severe skull and brain injury. The fracture results in separation of all facial bones of midface from base of skull at the level of nasofrontal suture line with simultaneous fracture of zygoma, maxilla and nasal bones. The fracture lines run posterior inferior to the optic foramen, across the lesser wing of sphenoid, to pterygomaxillary fissure and sphenopalatine foramen. The fracture also traverses the medial wall of orbit, to the superior orbital fissure, greater wing of sphenoid, zygomatic bone and zygomaticofrontal suture line. There is mobility of complete midface, which is detected at the frontonasal and

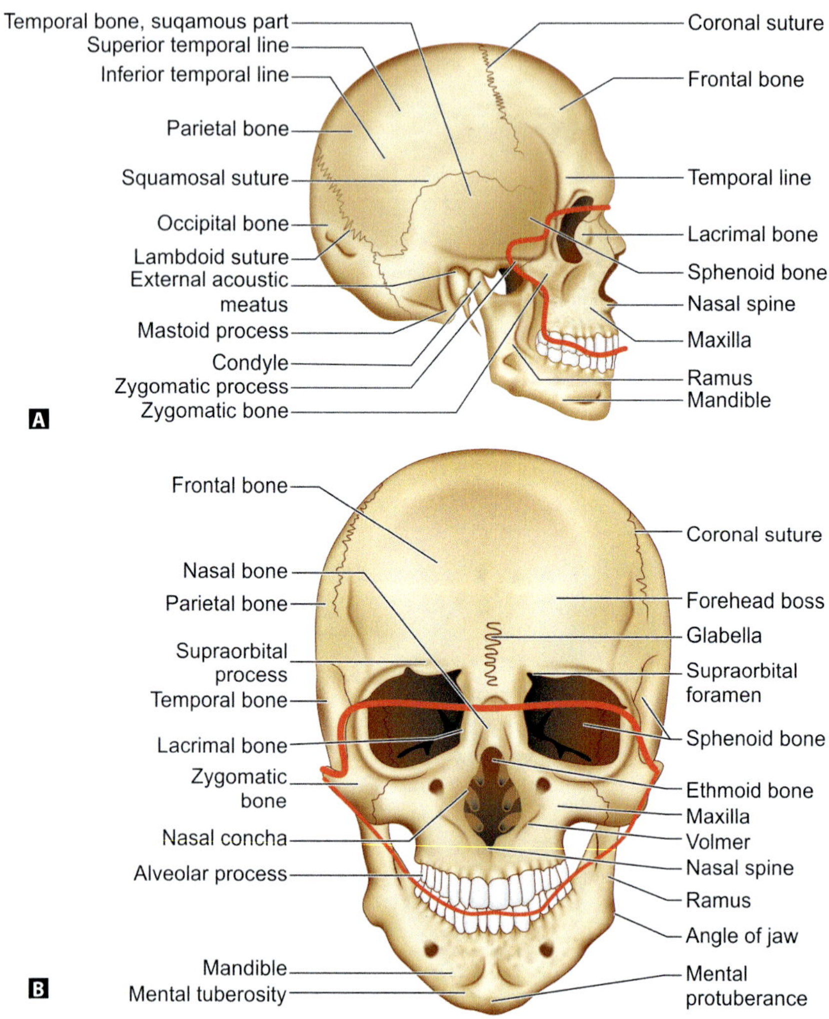

Figures 9.8A and B LeFort III or craniofacial disjunction or dislocation. (A) Lateral view; (B) Frontal view

frontozygomatic suture lines. The displacement is downward and backward along the base of skull imparting a dish face deformity and few may be associated with midline palatine fracture.

Lower Face

Fractures of the Mandible

The fractures of lower face involves the fractures of the mandible, which presents with several patterns and combinations of fracture and each is determined by the magnitude of the impact, the direction of the blow, the age of the patient, state of the jaws and condition of dentition. The weakest part of the mandible is the subcondylar region and is therefore the most common site of fractures.

The most usual combinations of mandibular fractures are as:

- More common
  - Fracture bilateral subcondylar regions
  - Fracture of body and opposite angle
  - Fracture of body with contralateral condyle
- Less common
  - Fracture of bilateral angle
  - Fracture of bilateral body
  - Comminuted fractures.

Rowe and Killey's Classification

- Fractures not involving the basal bone—are termed as dentoalveolar fractures
- Fractures involving the basal bone of the mandible subdivided into following:
  - Single unilateral
  - Double unilateral
  - Bilaterally
  - Multiple.

Dingman and Natvig's Classification by Anatomic Region

- Symphysis fractures
- Canine region fractures
- Body of mandible fractures
- Angle region fractures
- Coronoid region fractures
- Condyle fractures
- Dentoalveolar fractures.

The incidence of fractures of mandible as far as the sites are concerned is given below (Figure 9.9)

- Condylar
- Subcondylar
- Coronoid
- Angle
- Body
- Symphysis and parasymphysis.

Pathological Types of Mandibular Fracture

- Simple (closed fracture)—there is fracture without injury to skin or mucosal lining

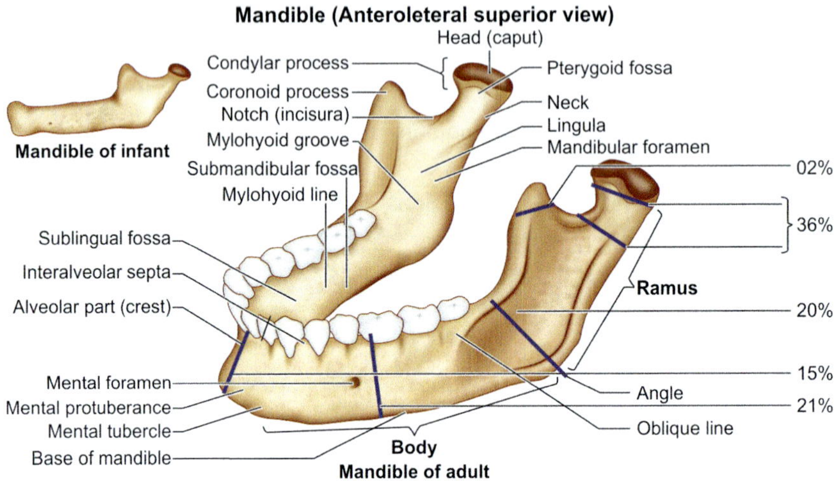

Figure 9.9 Parts of the mandible with incidence of proneness to fractures

- Compound (open fracture)—here the fracture communicates externally through skin or mucosal lining
- Multiple—two or more fractures
- Indirect—fracture site is distant from the site of injury
- Complex—the fracture may be single or compound with significant tissue injury.
- Comminuted—fracture with crushed bone
- Green stick—incomplete fracture in which one cortex is fractured and other cortex is intact
- Pathological—there is fracture from mild injury due to existing bone disease
- Impacted—after fracture one segment is driven into the other one
- Atrophic—fracture due severe atrophy of bone.

Displacements in Different Types of Mandibular Fractures (Figures 9.10 and 9.11)

- Fracture condyle—there occurs anteromedial rotation of condyle secondary to the pull due to lateral pterygoid muscles
- Fracture angle of mandible: The factors responsible for the pull are:
  - Posterior segment is pulled to medially, upward and forward by masseter, medial pterygoid and temporalis muscles
  - Direction of the fracture lies in vertical or horizontal plane.

When the muscle pull resists the displacement of the fragments then the fracture line is considered favorable fractures. When the muscle pull distracts the displacement of the fragments then the fracture line is considered unfavorable fractures. Therefore,

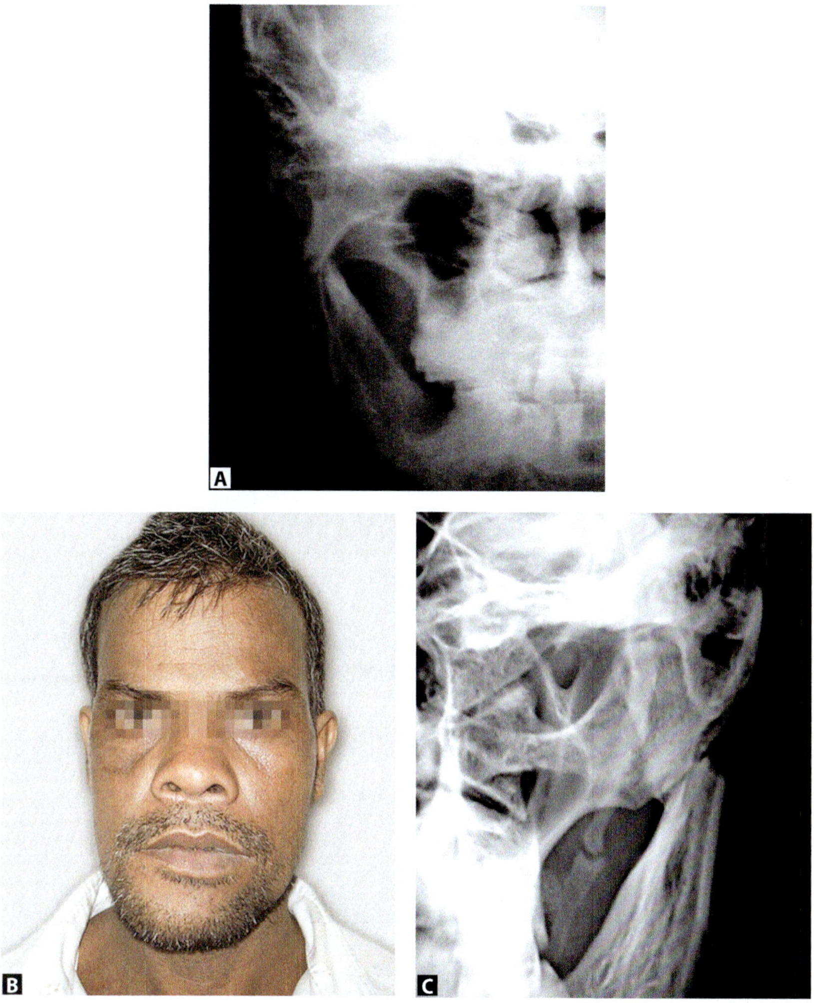

Figures 9.10A to C Left subcondylar fracture

- Fractures running forward from lingual to buccal aspect resist medial displacement and are known as vertically favorable fractures
- Fractures running backward from buccal to lingual aspect lead to easy displacement—lingually and are known as vertically unfavorable fractures
- Fractures running from superior border of mandible forward to inferior margin resist upward displacement—horizontally favorable fractures
- Fractures running from opposite to the above distract the fragments more and are known as horizontally unfavorable fractures.

▪ Body of mandible: There is medial displacement of posterior segment due to mylohyoid muscle pull.

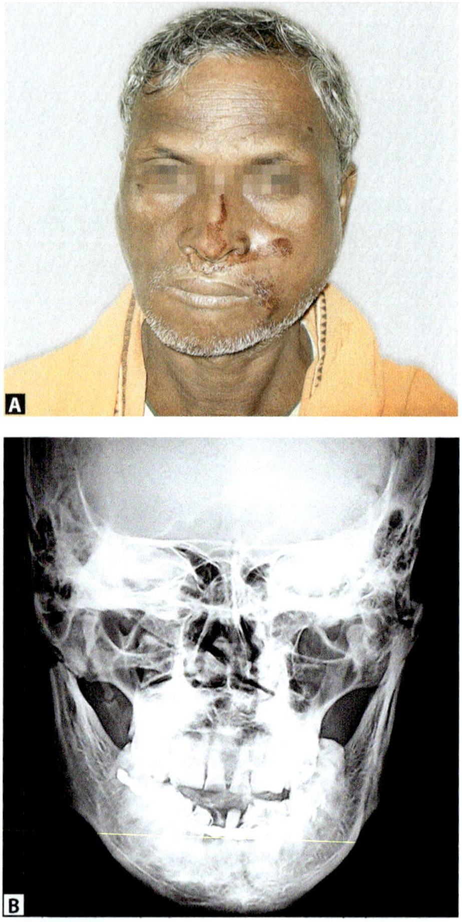

Figures 9.11A and B Bilateral subcondylar fracture

MANAGEMENT PROTOCOL OF THE FACIOMAXILLARY INJURIES

Primary Survey and Management

In maxillofacial injuries, as well as in all aspects of trauma management, the primary aim is to establish the patient's vital functions first than to go for immediate definite clinical examination of the patient as soon as the patient reports to the out-patient department, as the maxillofacial injuries can endanger the airway and are often associated with brain damage, chest injuries, and visceral injuries especially in high force impacts as it is in road traffic accidents. Therefore, in maxillofacial injury, first ensure the adequate airway and ventilation; look for abdomen, thorax and neck regions; assess the level of consciousness and also look for whether there is any feature of shock.

All the protocols for evaluation and management of an endangered patient should be maintained as per ABCDE (airway, breathing, circulation, disability/ drugs, exposure or environment control) of primary care. The primary care is the rapid identification and treatment of life-threatening injuries such as airway obstruction, tension or open pneumothorax, flail chest, massive hemorrhage and cardiac tamponade. It should be quick and complete. Further detailed examination for definitive treatment of facial injury must take the secondary place.

The Need for Airway

It is carefully considered in both the conscious and comatose patients in those, who have compromised airway such as posterior displacement of tongue secondary to the mandibular fractures or posteroinferior displacement of the maxilla with middle third of face injuries. Non-surgical procedures for maintaining the airways like (1) Chin lift, (2) Jaw thrust, (3) Oropharyngeal airway, (4) Nasopharyngeal airway, (5) Orotracheal intubation, and (6) Nasotracheal intubation may be required.

If no cervical spine injury is suspected, attempts to open the airway may be made carefully with head tilt or chin lift maneuver and avoid over extension by pulling the patient in neutral position for infants and sniffing position for children. In case, if a cervical spine injury is suspected, the jaw thrust technique is preferred. Middle third fracture may be reduced immediately by hooking the fingers of one hand around the posterior margin of the patient's hard palate and pulling the displaced jaw forward. These patients may progress rapidly to severe airway compromising state due to oropharyngeal edema.

Therefore, middle third facial fractures as well as paradoxical chest movement due to flail chest require endotracheal intubation (orotracheal intubation/ nasotracheal intubation). Blood, vomitus, tooth fragments, and foreign body may obstruct the airway and, clearance of all debris is a priority.

A displaced tongue secondary to comminuted anterior mandibular fracture may also compromise the airway, which may be taken care of. If the patient's tongue or lower jaws has fallen backwards, then put some suture or towel clip through it and gently pull it forwards. The patient is allowed to lie down on his side. If patient's soft palate has been driven onto his tongue then hook your fingers around the back of his hard palate and then, the middle of the face is gently pulled upward and forwards so that the airway is restored properly. However, if fracture segments are impacted and it failed to reduce, then tracheostomy is essentially needed to save the life. This disimpaction is done by gripping the patient's alveolus with Rowe's forceps and is rocked to disimpact the maxillary fragments. If the patient has severe jaw injury with much tissue loss then transport the patient on the stretcher on his front in prone position, while the head slightly hanging from the end of the stretcher and forehead is supported by bandages between the handles of it.

If the patient's nose is more severely injured and there is bleeding, then the blood is sucked out and an oropharyngeal airway or nasopharyngeal tube is inserted down one side, and that is regularly sucked out with a suction machine to prevent blockage. But however, if reduction of middle third face is not possible immediately; if severe posterior third bleeding is not controllable edema of glottis following neck injury, then a tracheostomy should immediately be required under local anesthesia and a cuffed PVC tracheostomy tube is put.

Control of Bleeding and Maintenance of Circulation

Origin of hemorrhage may be detected and managed. Shock is due to hemorrhage and mostly due to trauma to internal structures rather than facial injury. Nasal bleeding can be controlled by adrenaline nasal packing. Other source of bleeding may be searched and must be stopped. Circulation should be maintained. The patient's level of consciousness, skin color and character of pulse will provide regarding his or her status. In injury, with no sources of external bleeding evident and patient in shock then a probable cause of bleeding, from internal organs like thorax, abdomen, retroperitoneum or from thigh or femur fracture may be sought for.

Assessment of Head Injury

After restoring adequate airway, circulation and establishing good hemostatic status, assessment of head injury is carried out, which is usually recorded by Glasgow Coma Score.

Glasgow Coma Score (GCS)

The GCS is scored between 3 and 15, 3 being the worst and 15, the best. It is composed of three parameters: best eye response, best verbal response, and best motor response, as follows (Table 9.2):

- Best Eye Response[4]
  - No eye opening
  - Eye opening to pain
  - Eye opening to verbal command
  - Eyes open spontaneously
- Best Verbal Response[5]
  - No verbal response
  - Incomprehensible sounds
  - Inappropriate words
  - Confused
  - Orientated

Table 9.2 Glasgow Coma Score for pediatrics[29]

Characters	*Scoring*
Best Motor Response (M)—6 grades Apply varied painful stimulus: Trapezius squeeze, earlobe pinch, supra-orbital pressure, sternal rub, nail-bed pressure, etc: 1. No response to pain 2. Extensor posturing to pain: The stimulus causes limb extension (abduction, internal rotation of shoulder, pronation of forearm, wrist extension)—decerebrate posture 3. Abnormal flexor response to pain: Stimulus causes abnormal flexion of the limbs (adduction of arm, internal rotation of shoulder, pronation of forearm, wrist flexion)—decorticate posture 4. Withdraws to pain: Pulls limb away from painful stimulus. Infant: Withdraws from pain 5. Localizing response to pain: Purposeful movements towards changing painful stimuli is a 'localizing' response. Infant: Withdraws from touch 6. Obeying command: The patient does simple things you ask (beware of accepting a grasp reflex in this category). Infant: Moves spontaneously or purposefully.	
Best Verbal Response (V)—5 grades Record best level of speech. If patient is intubated, a "derived verbal score" is calculated via a linear regression prediction. 1. No verbal response 2. Incomprehensible speech: Moaning but no words. Infant: Inconsolable, agitated 3. Inappropriate speech: Random or exclamatory articulated speech, but no conversational exchange Infant: Inconsistantly inconsolable moaning 4. Confused conversation: Patient responds to questions in a conversational manner but some disorientation and confusion. Infant: Cries but consolable, inappropriate interactions 5. Orientated: Patient 'knows who he is, where he is and why, the year, season, and month, Infant: Smiles, orientated to sounds, follows objects, interacts.	
Best Eye Response (E)—4 grades 1. No eye opening 2. Opening to response to pain to limbs as above 3. Eye opening in response any speech (or shout, not necessarily request to open eyes) 4. Spontaneous eye opening.	
Glasgow Coma Scale Score (max 15):	(Derived Verbal score:)
Interpretation of Symptoms: (Severe: 8 or less; Moderate: 9–12; Mild: 13 or more)	

- Best Motor Response[6]
  - No motor response
  - Extension to pain
  - Flexion to pain
  - Withdrawal from pain
  - Localizing pain
  - Obeys commands.

Note that the phrase 'GCS of 11' is essentially meaningless, and it is important to break the figure down into its components, such as E3V3M5 = GCS 11.

A Coma Score of 13 or higher correlates with a mild brain injury; 9 to 12 is a moderate injury and 8 or less, a severe brain injury.

This gives a reliable, objective way of recording the conscious state of a person. It can be used by medical and nursing staff for initial and continuing assessment. It has value in predicting ultimate outcome. Three types of response are independently assessed and are recorded on an appropriate chart (and the overall score is made by summing the scores). The calculator has been adapted to estimate the Glasgow verbal score from the Glasgow eye and motor scores in intubated patients. There is a pediatric Glasgow Coma Scale applicable to infants too young to speak and the equivalent infant responses are given in the various sections of this chapter.

Examination of Eyes

Inspection

Look for penetrating injuries, corneal abrasion, and dislocation of lens, laceration involving the lacrimal apparatus, exophthalmos or enophthalmos or fat protruding from the globe. In conscious patient, visual acuity, ophthalmoscopic examination for retinal damage and ischemia, light reflexes, external eye movements, interpupillary distance, pupillary size and shape, etc. are to be inspected. Evert the eyelids and check for foreign bodies or laceration. Raccoon eyes (also known in the UK as panda eyes) or periorbital ecchymosis is a sign of basal skull fracture.[30] Bilateral subconjunctival hemorrhage occurs when damage at the time of a facial fracture tears the meninges and causes the venous sinuses to bleed into the arachnoid villi and the cranial sinuses. Pain and swelling are the most common signs and symptoms of a black eye. Raccoon eyes may be accompanied by Battle's sign, an ecchymosis behind the ear. If the patient has massive proptosis, it may be due to severe retrobulbar hemorrhage due to fracture of skull base causing blindness, compressing his optic nerve. Make a small incision at outer canthus, take a hemostat and push onto the incision. This may prevent his blindness. A displacement of eyeball downwards and inwards indicates herniation of the contents through the floor of the orbit into maxillary sinus or a fracture of zygomatico-frontomaxillary complex. Examine for the presence of diplopia by separating the eyelids. Other signs of more serious injury are double vision, loss of sight, loss of consciousness, inability to move the eye, blood or clear fluid from the nose or the ears, blood on the surface of the eye itself and persistent headache. Examine the anterior chamber for presence of blood. Tenderness on palpation on medial orbital area signifies damage to the nasoethmoidal complex. On palpation, examine for forced duction (test) to see for the avulsion of the medial canthal ligament that produces an abnormal slant of palpebral fissure, if positive. Also, perform traction test for status of medial canthal ligament attachment by grasping the lower eyelid and pulling against its medial attachment. If the test gives of then there is obvious medial canthal disruption.

Examination of Nose

Unilateral epistaxis without presence of direct nasal injury may indicate fracture of maxillary antrum. Look for the facial asymmetry; compare one side of the face with other side and also find whether nose or face is flattened. Inspect for telecanthus and palpate for tenderness or dislocation. Inspect the nasal septum for hematoma, deviation, mucosal laceration, fracture or CSF leak. Perform bimanual nasal palpation test by pressing the anesthetized nasal cavity with a finger against medial orbital rim and simultaneously pressing the medial canthus. If bone moves, then the nasoethmoidal complex is fractured. Put a hand on anterior nasal bridge and another on bridge of nose and feel for mobility. If only teeth move, then it is LeFort I fracture and if both nose and maxilla move together, then it may be LeFort II or III fractures.

Examination of Ears

Inspect the ear canal for laceration, CSF leak, integrity of tympanic membrane hemotympanum, perforation or mastoid area ecchymosis (Battle's Sign).

Examination of Tongue and Oral Cavity

Inspect for intraoral laceration, ecchymosis and swelling. Bimanually, palpate for mandible for its mobility, integrity, tenderness and crepitus. Palpate each tooth individually for movement, pain, gingival and intraoral bleeding, tears and crepitus. Perform the tongue blade test by asking the patient to bite hard on a tongue blade and if the patient cannot bite, then the jaw is fractured.

Miscellaneous Approach

- Do not move the damaged or broken facial bones at first instance, otherwise it will make the situation worse
- Wound decontamination and debridement
- Wound assessment—for assessing the injury to the major blood vessels, nerves, ligaments, joints, bones or internal organs

- Wound exploration and closure—after the patient is all stable
- X-ray of chest to exclude any thoracic injury.

Medical Therapy

- Antibiotics—for fractures with dural tears or CSF leaks, the drug of choice is vancomycin and ceftazidime. For comminuted sinus fractures, the drug of choice is amoxicillin-clavulanic. For facial laceration, the drug of choice is ceftriaxone and for oral cavity laceration, the drug of choice is clindamycin
- Pain management
- General medical therapy—administration of oxygen, intravenous fluids, blood transfusion and tetanus prophylaxis.

SECONDARY SURVEY AND CLINICAL FEATURES OF THE FACIOMAXILLARY INJURIES

After the patient is stabilized from the initial airway distress, hemorrhage or shock, then the secondary survey or final assessment of the injury to detect the type, depth, extent and degree of injuries is done for further management. The optimal time for definitive treatment is between 5th to 8th post-traumatic day during which the inflammatory swelling would have been subsided and patient's general medical condition would have been improved. And it also allows sufficient time to assess the fracture, to make splints if required. Wash the face with warm water or saline water to remove the caked blood for better assessment of injuries.

CLINICAL FEATURES OF INDIVIDUAL FRACTURES

- **Frontal bone fractures:**
  - Disruption or crepitus of the supraorbital rims
  - Subcutaneous emphysema
  - Paresthesia of supraorbital and supratrochlear nerve distribution
  - Soft tissue edema over the frontal region, periorbital ecchymosis and edema
  - Soft tissue contusion or laceration over frontal sinus area
  - Epistaxis or CSF rhinorrhea.
- **Nasal bone fractures:**

  Isolated nasal fractures are the most commonly seen fractures in facial trauma. However, these may be associated with severe midfacial trauma involving the naso-orbito-ethmoidal (NOE) complex, frontal sinuses, the orbitozygomatic complex or isolated nasal bone fractures. The fractures of nasal bones are classified into three following classes:

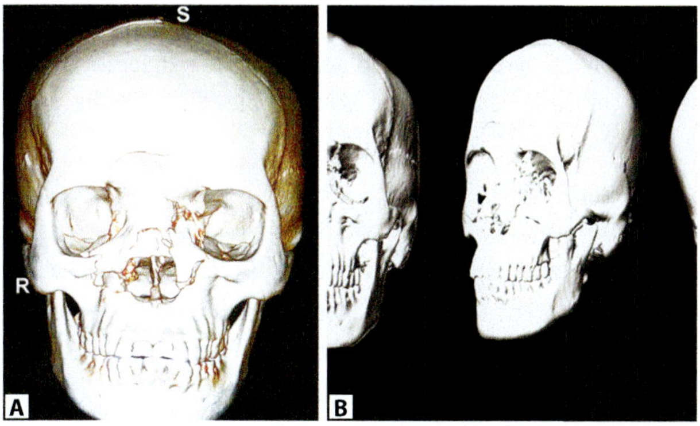

Figures 9.12A and B A 3-D reconstruced CT scan of skull showing naso-orbito-ethmoidal fractures

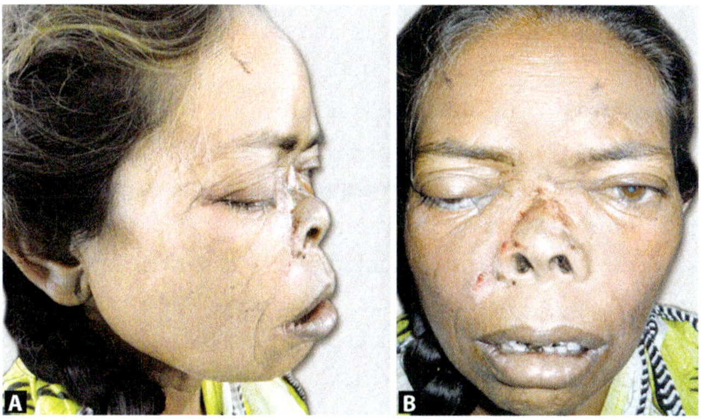

Figures 9.13A and B Naso-orbito-ethmoidal fracture of same patient: pig-like appearance

Class–I or Chevallet fracture: Here, the fracture line runs through the nasal bone and proximal part of the quadrilateral cartilage the vertical fracture that runs on the septum is known as Chevallet fracture.

Class–II fracture: This involves the fracture of nasal bone, perpendicular plate of ethmoid, vomer and quadrilateral cartilage.

Class–III fracture: When the fracture extends to include the ethmoid labyrinth, then perpendicular plate along with ethmoid air cells are pulled backward causing a pig, like appearance with forward facing nostril and saddling (Figures 9.12 and 9.13).

The fracture of nasal bone may be complicated with, deviated nasal septum, bleeding, saddling, CSF leak and orbital complications like hypertelorism, diplopia, damage to lacrimal sac and nasolacrimal duct, dacryocystitis and blindness.

- **Orbital fracture:**
    - A black eye, with swelling and black and blue discoloration around the injured eye; possible redness and areas of bleeding on the white of the eye and on the inner lining of the eyelids
    - Double vision, decreased vision or blurred vision
    - Difficulty in looking up, down, right or left
    - Abnormal position of the eye (either bulging out of its socket or sunken in)
    - Numbness in the forehead, eyelids, cheek, upper lip or upper teeth on the same side as the injured eye, possibly related to nerve damage caused by the fracture
    - A puffy accumulation of air under the skin near the eye, usually a sign that the fracture has broken through the wall of a sinus cavity, particularly the maxillary sinus
    - Swelling and deformity of the cheek or forehead, with an obvious dent over the area of broken bone
    - An abnormally flat-looking cheek and possibly severe pain in the cheek when you attempt to open your mouth.
- **Orbital floor fracture or blow-out fractures:**

    The orbital floor fracture can present with periorbital edema, crepitus, ecchymosis, enophthalmos, ocular injury, anesthesia or paresthesia of cheek and upper gum on affected side, lateral and upward gaze dysfunction due to medial and lateral rectus entrapment, diplopia as patient gazes upward due to entrapment of inferior rectus muscle. In trap-door type, orbital floor fracture leading to entrapment may cause nausea, vomiting, bradycardia, hypothermia and pain in the eye (oculocardiac reflex).
- **Zygomaticomaxillary complex fractures:**

    The zygomaticomaxillary complex fractures can present in the following ways:

    Orbital features
    - Periorbital swelling
    - Ecchymosis
    - Subconjunctival hemorrhage
    - Diplopia secondary to extraocular dysfunction
    - Enophthalmos
    - Paresthesia in infraorbital nerve distribution
    - Palpable depression of orbital rim and zygomatic arch
    - Step defect—palpated along the infraorbital rim or zygomaticomaxillary suture.

    Nasal and zygomatic features
    - Loss and flattening of zygomatic body prominence
    - Epistaxis
    - Tenderness of frontozygomatic suture line
    - Trismus due to impingement of coronoid process of mandible

- Intraoral ecchymosis epistaxis
- Flame sign may be present due to dispersion and depression of the lateral canthal tendon.

▪ **Zygomatic arch fracture:**

This fracture exhibits a palpable defect over the area involved, with pain on palpation. There is limitation of movement of mandible.

▪ **Maxillary factures:**

The maxillary facture are more common in adults than in children. The maxilla in children is proportionately smaller and denser than the adults with a relative lack of sinus development. Therefore, isolated displacement of part of or all of the maxillary complex is rare. In children, however, when fracture occurs, then there is generally more extensive craniofacial injuries with skull fracture, CSF rhinorrhea and cervical spine injuries.

Clinical features of maxillary fractures are as follows:

- Bilateral periorbital or circumorbital swelling and ecchymosis
- Bilateral subconjunctival hemorrhage
- Facial deformity, asymmetry, flattening or elongation
- Intraorbital paresthesia
- Palpable step deformity of infraorbital margins and tenderness at fronto-zygomatic sutures
- Malocclusion
- CSF rhinorrhea
- Mobility of maxilla at different levels usually representing three recognizable patterns of fractures namely LeFort—I, II, and III
  - LeFort—I: Maxilla is mobile to the level of the base of the nose with a stable upper midface
  - LeForte—II: Maxilla and nose are mobile as one unit with the movement detected at fronto-orbital rims
  - LeForte—III Mobility of complete midface with movement detected at the frontonasal and frontozygomatic sutures
- Midline palatal fractures result in independent movement of the right and left maxilla, laceration of palatine bone and floating palate and teeth.

▪ **Mandibular factures:**

Body, angle and smphysis (Figures 9.14 and 9.15)

- Step deformity—palpable externally and orally
- Asymmetry of lower dental arch and derangement of occlusion
- Pain, paradoxical movement and crepitus on distribution of fracture segment
- Hematoma in buccal sulcus or floor of mouth
- Blood stained saliva
- Anesthesia in mental nerve distribute.

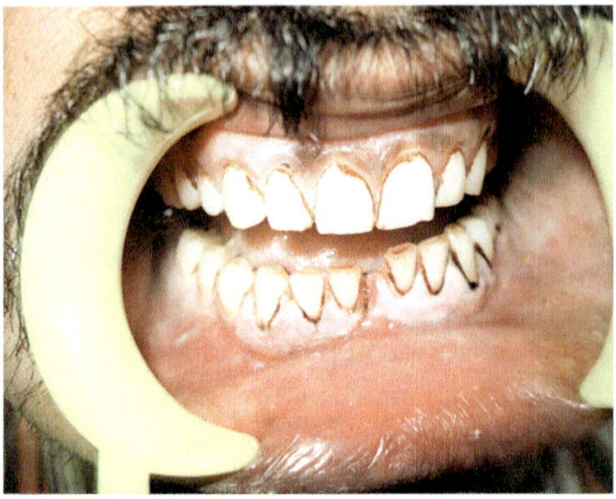

Figure 9.14 Symphysis fracture of mandible

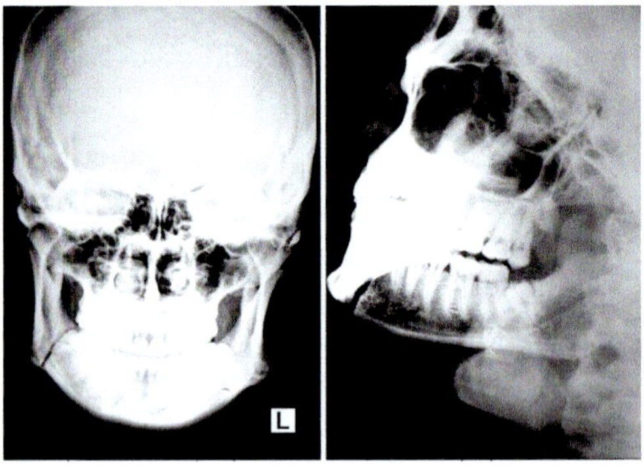

Figure 9.15 Symphysis and angle fractures

- **Condyle fracture:**
  - Temporomandibular joint tenderness
  - Trismus
  - The deviation of the jaw towards the injured side on opening of mouth
  - Inability to move the mandible to the side opposite to the injury
  - The deviation of the jaw towards the injured side on rest with anterior open bite secondary to the gagging
  - Symmetrical anterior open bite on bilateral fractures of the necks of the condyle.

INVESTIGATIONS AND WORK UP

Laboratory Study

Complete blood count every 4 hours to follow hemoglobin and hematocrit; sequential multiple analysis of 20 chemical constituents (SMA-20); blood grouping and cross matching, coagulation studies and tests for hepatitis and HIV are to be done routinely.

CSF study of nasal discharge, if suspected.

Imaging Study

- *Upper face:* The study of choice is axial or coronal CT scan. Alternate studies include X-rays of skull in Water's view
- *Mid face:* The study of choice is axial or coronal CT scan. Alternate studies include X-rays of skull in Water's view, posteroanterior and submentovertex views and occlusal views
- *Lower face:* The study of choice is pantomographic X-rays. Alternate studies include X-rays of posteroanterior view, right and left lateral oblique views of mandible, elongated Towne projection and occlusal X-rays. For condylar fracture, CT scanning is strongly recommended.

  Three-dimensional CT reconstruction, if possible.

For temporomandibular joint injury and CSF leak—MRI is the choice of investigation.

DEFINITIVE TREATMENTS

Frontal Bone Fracture

- Nondisplaced anterior sinus wall fracture—observation and antibiotics
- Displaced anterior sinus wall fracture with severe comminution and mucosal injury—bone grafting and frontal sinus obliteration by otolaryngologist, maxillofacial surgeon or plastic surgeon
- Nondisplaced posterior sinus wall with CSF leak—may be observed for 5–7 days and frontal sinus obliteration is done, should the CSF leak persists
- Displaced fractures of posterior wall without CSF leak with mild comminution—osteoplastic flap and sinus obliteration surgery
- Displaced fractures of posterior wall without CSF leak with more than 30% comminution—removal of posterior table by neurosurgeon—cranialization
- Displaced fractures of posterior wall with CSF leak with minimal to mild comminution—sinus obliteration surgery
- Displaced fractures of posterior wall with CSF leak with moderate to severe comminution—cranialization.

Orbital Floor Fracture

Orbital floor fractures require consultation with an ophthalmologist, otorhinolaryngologist, oral and maxillofacial surgeon and plastic surgeon depending upon requirements. Maximum window period for repair of orbital floor is 2 weeks.

However, patients with oculocardiac reflex should undergo immediate exploration of the orbit.

For isolated fracture of the orbital floor, transconjunctival incision without canthotomy is ideal, whereas for major isolated fracture of the orbital floor subciliary approach is indicated and repair is usually done with autologous bone graft or alloplastic material. Indications for major fracture repair are:

- Defect of floor >50%
- Enophthalmos >2 mm due to herniation in blow out fractures
- Diplopia on upward/downward gaze
- Positive forced duction test within 30% of primary gaze CT confirmation of fracture.

Nasal Bone Fractures

Fracture of isolated nasal bone is repaired by closed reduction of nasal bone and of septum by otolaryngologist within 5–7 days after swelling is subsided. The support is given by intranasal packing and extranasal splinting.

Nasoethmoidal Fractures

This requires a multispecialist approach.

Zygomatic Arch Fractures

Many of the zygomatic fractures do not need reduction in view of real risk of iatrogenic blindness following treatment in minimal defect. Reduction of zygoma can only be done by open reduction.

Temporal Fossa Approach

A skin incision is given just behind the hairline anterosuperior to the pinna and that is developed through the fascia. A Rowe elevator is used to reduce the zygomatic arch while not pressing on the parietal bone.

Transcutaneous Approach

The temporary fixation may be applied by packing the maxillary antrum through Caldwell-Luc's approach or by silicon wedge supporting the lateral antral wall or a Folley catheter intranasally.

Zygomaticomaxillary Complex Fractures

Otolaryngologists, plastic surgeon and oral and maxillofacial surgeons should be consulted for this type of fractures. The standard treatment is open reduction and fixation with mini plates.

Maxillary Fractures

Principle

Otolaryngologists, plastic surgeon and oral and maxillofacial surgeons should be consulted for this type of fractures. A principle in all LeFort fractures is to re-establish the premorbid dental occlusion. Portions of the pterygoid plates and associated musculature are still attached to the posterior portion of the maxilla, so passive mobilization of the fracture can be difficult. In isolated maxillary fractures, the stable cranium above and occlusal plate below provide sources of stable fixation. If available, dental cast, stereolithographic models, and/or premorbid photographs may be useful guides for treatment.

Preoperative Preparation

The patient should be informed about the risks and possible complications of the procedure, possibility of temporary or permanent paresthesia, cerebrospinal fluid leak, meningitis, sinus infection or mucocele, anosmia, malocclusion, infection of implants, osteomyelitis, malunion or nonunion, external deformity, plate exposure, tooth injury and the possible need for additional surgery due to treatment of maxillomandibular fixation (MMF).

Operative Plan and Procedures

The MMF is typically performed with arch bars and stainless steel 25 or 26 gauge interdental wires. For edentulous patients, surgical splints or dentures secured to the underlying bone with screws or with circummandibular and circumzygomatic wiring serve as the basis of stabilization. The method of treatment is open reduction and interaxillary fixation (which is not used now a days), followed by rigid fixation at pyriform rims and zygomaticomaxillary buttress. Internal fixation may be indicated with transosseous wire fixation, miniplate fixation, or use of resorbable plate and screw fixation. Nondisplaced, stable fractures with normal occlusion is managed, conservatively. Displaced or unstable fractures are reduced and stabilized to restore functional occlusion, facial contour and symmetry.

In general, treatment for LeFort and alveolar fractures are external and internal fixation. Method applied for external fixation are, plastic head cap, levant frame, box frame and facial transfixation and for internal fixation are internal wire suspension, direct wiring, and miniplates.

LeFort I Fractures

For stable, nondisplaced LeFort I fractures, MMF alone may suffice to provide stable restoration of bony support. Unstable fractures require an additional means of fixation. The method of choice for fixation is through miniplates placed via an open approach. A gingivolabial incision through mucosa 5–10 mm labial to the apex of the sulcus is given (Figures 9.16A and B).

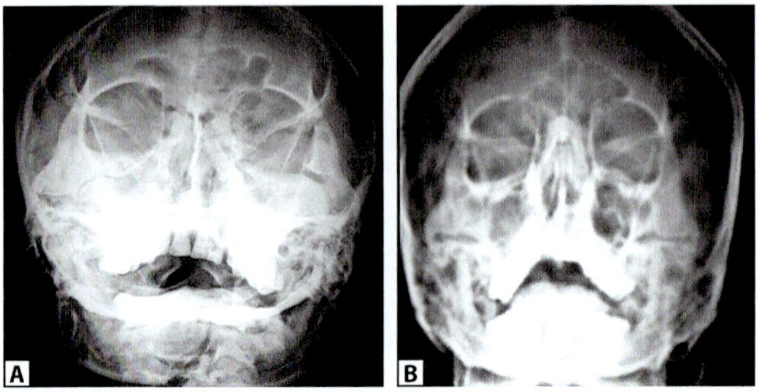

Figures 9.16A and B LeFort I fractures on AP view of X-rays

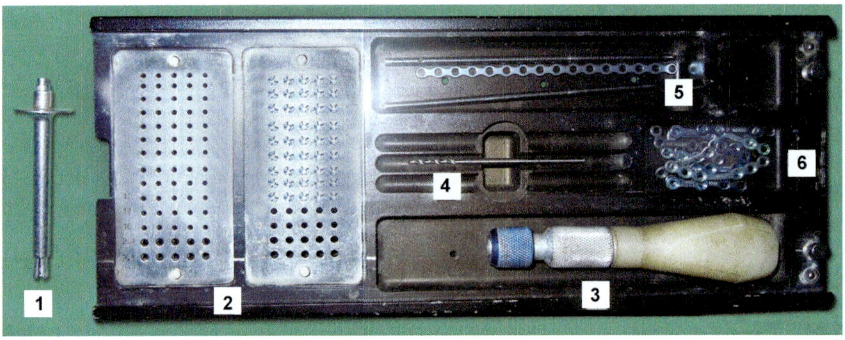

Figure 9.17 A complete tool box containing (1 and 3), screw driver, (2) screw holder, (4) drill bit, (5 and 6) mini and long plates

Incision is extended down to alveolar bone from one molar region to the other. Elevate the periosteum superiorly to expose the fracture lines not injuring the infraorbital nerve. Expose the nasomaxillary and zygomaticomaxillary buttresses, piriform aperture and premaxilla and nasal spine. Contour vertically oriented miniplates using a malleable template to span the fracture line. Plating with low-profile titanium plates secured with monocortical self-tapping screws across the nasomaxillary and zygomaticomaxillary buttresses are sufficient. In an alternative, a 25 or 26 gauge wire is looped around the temporal aspect of the zygomatic arch retrieved intraorally and tightened to an intermediate wire loop connected to the arch bar (Figures 9.17 to 9.19).

LeFort II Fractures (Figure 9.20)

Here, initial exposure is same as LeFort I and extension of exposure is superiorly done for adequate exploration of the orbital rim. This is achieved through subciliary or transconjunctival incisions. More extensive degloving of the soft

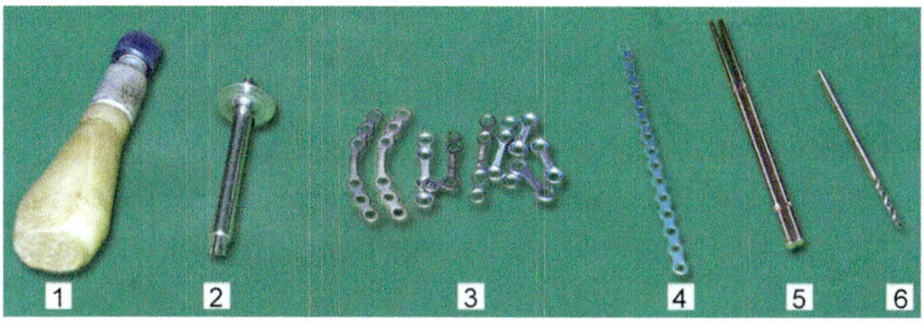

Figure 9.18 Complete tool box containing (1 and 2) screw driver, (3 and 4) mini and long plates (5 and 6), parts of the drill bits

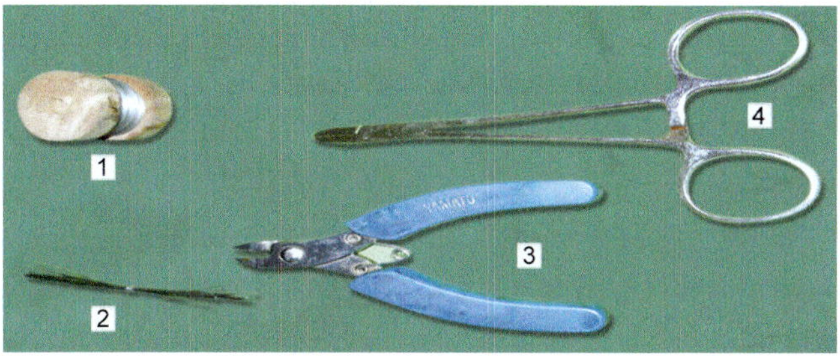

Figure 9.19 A tool set containing (1 and 2)—stainless steel wire, (3)—wire cutter, (4)—wire twister

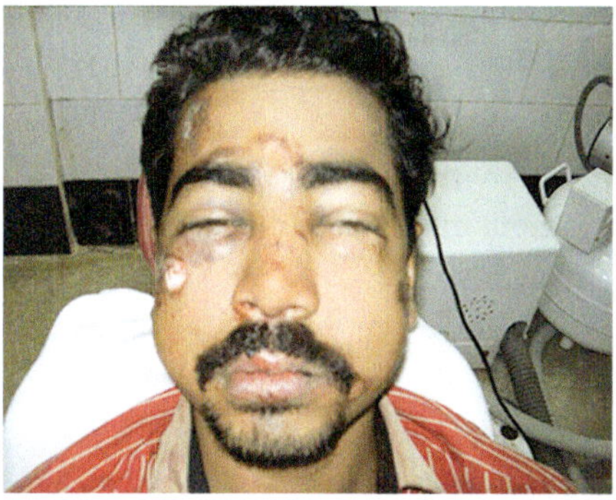

Figure 9.20 LeFort II fracture

tissue envelope through exposure of the piriform aperture and frontomaxillary region is facilitated by columellar-septal transfixion incisions. The pyramidal free maxillary segment is stabilized to the intact zygoma. Fixation is completed directly using noncompression miniplates. Accurate contouring of the plates using malleable templates is important for reduction and fixation. Monocortical, self-tapping screws are ideal. Alternative to miniplates is interosseous wiring.

LeFort III Fractures

In LeFort III fractures, the mobile segments of bone are stabilized to the stable mandible below and cranium above. Initially, the maxilla must be disimpacted and MMF implemented. Soft tissue incisions is made in the same locations as for LeFort II fractures. Lateral brow incisions, glabellar fold incisions, or bicoronal scalp flaps can be used for additional exposure to the frontozygomatic buttress. Miniplate fixation is currently the most reliable and rigid method. Malleable templates, accurate contouring of plates, and monocortical, self-tapping screws are used. Bilateral zygomaticofrontal fixation is sufficient. Additional points of fixation like, nasomaxillary, nasofrontal, inferior orbital rim, zygomatic arch may be required.

Interosseous wiring and suspension wiring have been described for LeFort III fractures but are less reliable. Extra skeletal fixation is not usually necessary for simple LeFort fractures.

Mandibular Fractures (Figures 9.21A and B)

Different methods are (Figures 9.22 to 9.26):

- Reduction
  - Closed reduction technique
    - Intermaxillary fixation
    - External pin fixation
  - Open reduction technique
    - Transosseous wiring
    - Compression plates
- Fixation or immobolization
  - Osteosynthesis without intermaxillary fixation
    - Compression plates
    - Non-compression plates
    - Miniplates
    - Lag screws
    - Resorbable plates and screws
  - Intermaxillary fixation
    - Bonded brackets
    - Dental wiring
    - Arch bars
    - Cap splints
  - Intermaxillary fixation with osteosynthesis
    - Transosseous wiring
    - Circumferential external pin wiring
    - External transfixation.

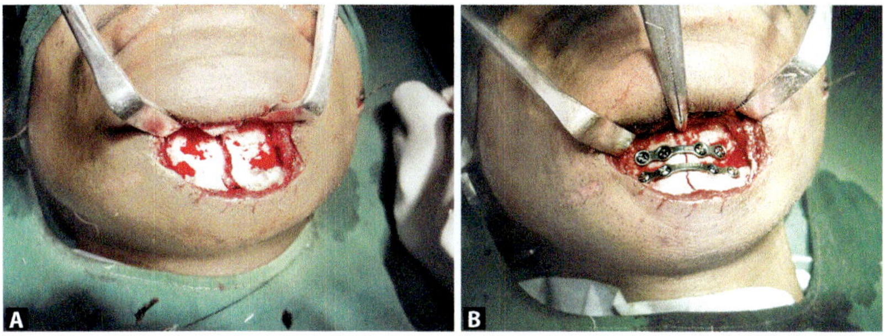

Figures 9.21A and B Symphysis fracture of mandible with platings

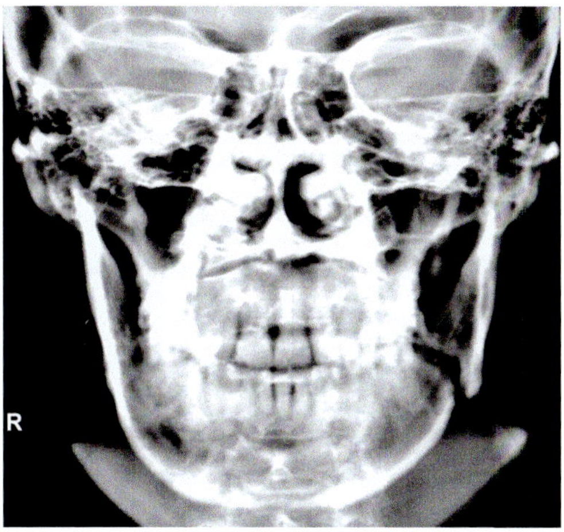

Figure 9.22 Digital X-rays of skull and mandible showing fracture of angle of mandible in left

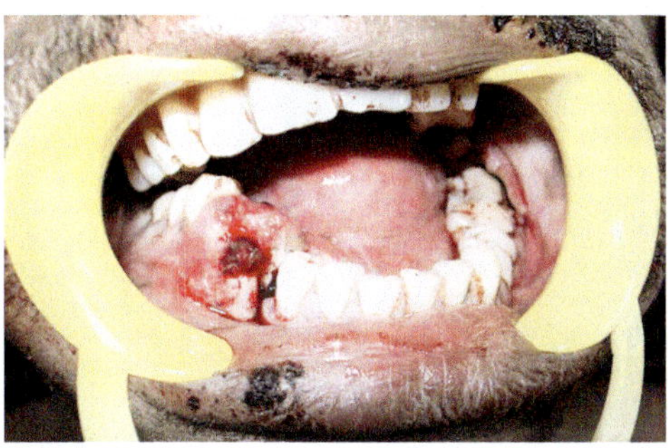

Figure 9.23 Parasymphysis fracture of mandible

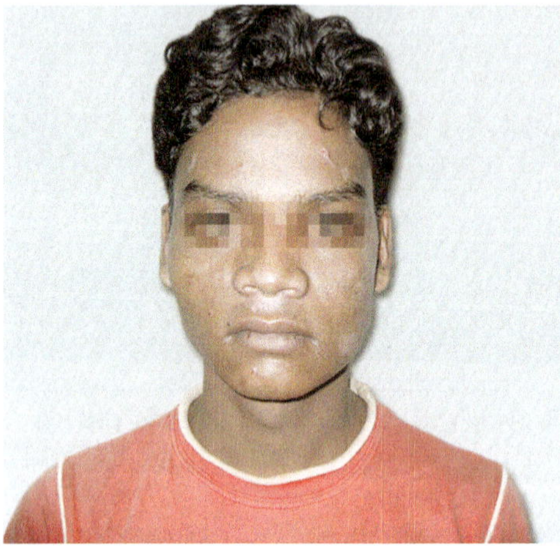

Figure 9.24 Fracture of angle of mandible in left mandible and zygoma

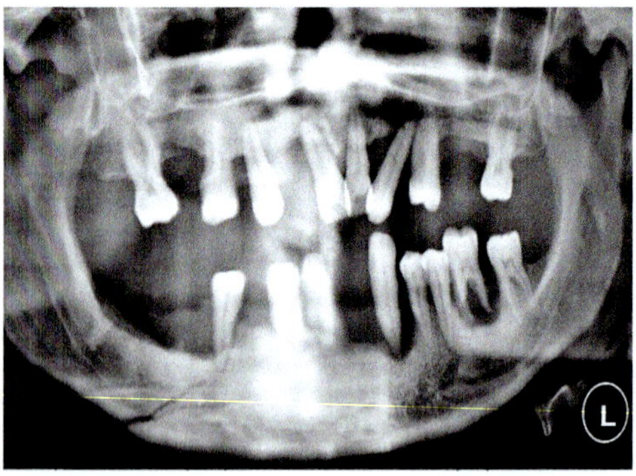

Figure 9.25 Orthopantomogram showing fracture of mandible

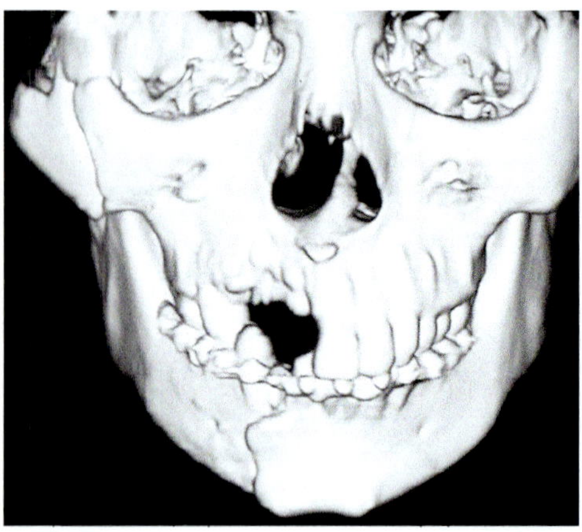

Figure 9.26 Three-dimension reconstructed CT showing fracture of mandible

COMPLICATIONS IN SURGERY OF MAXILLOFACIAL INJURIES

- Aspiration, airway compression, scars, permanent facial deformity, nerve damage
- Chronic sinusitis, infection, malnutrition, weight loss, nonunion or malunion of fractures
- Malocclusion or hemorrhage.

REFERENCES

1. Gassner R, Tuli T, Hachi O, Rudisch A, Ulmer H. Cranio-maxilllofacial trauma: A 10 year review of 9543 cases with 21067 injuries. Craniomaxillofacial Surg. 2003;31:51-61.
2. Laskin DM, Best AM. Current trends in the treatment of maxillofacial injures in the United States. J Oral Maxillofacial Surg. 2000;58:207-15.
3. Beers MH, Berkow R (Eds). The Merck Manual of Diagnosis and Therapy. Whitehouse Station, NJ: Merck Research Laboratories. 2002.
4. Rana ZA, Khoso NA, Arsad O, Siddiqi KM. An assessment of maxillofacial injuries: A 5-year study of 2112 patients. Ann Pak Inst Med Sci. 2010;6(2):113-5.
5. Lida S, Hassfeld JF, Reuther T, Schweigert H, Klein J, et al. Maxillofacial fractures resulting from falls. J Craniomaxillofac Surg. 2003;31:278-83.
6. Bamjee Y, Lownie JF, Cleaton-Jones PE, Lownie MA. Maxillofacial injuries in a group of South Africans under 18 years of age. Br J Oral Maxillofacial Surg. 1996;34:298-302.
7. Bataineh AB. Etiology and incidence of maxillofacial fractures in north of Jordan. J Oral Surg Oral Med Oral Pathol. 1998;86:31.
8. Motamedi MH. An assessment of maxillofacial fractures; a 5-year study of 237 patients. J Oral Maxillofac Surg. 2003;61:61-4.
9. Subhasraj K, Nandkumar N, Ravindran. Review of maxillofacial injuries in Chennai, India; A study of 2748 cases. British Journal of Oral and Maxillofacial Surgery. 2007;45: 637-9.
10. Laski R, Ziccardi VB, Broder H, Janal M. Facial trauma; a recurrent disease? The potential role of disease prevention. J Oral Maxillofac Surg. 2004;62:685-8.
11. Schaftenarr E, Bastiaens GJ, Simon EN, Morkx MA. Presentation and management of maxillofacial trauma in Dar Es Salaam, Tanzania East. Afro Med J. 2009;86(6):254-8.
12. Cheema F Amin. Incidence and causes of maxillofacial skeletal injuries at the Mayo hospital in Lahore, Pakistan British Journal of Oral and Maxillofacial Surgery. 2006; 44:232-4.
13. Leles R et al. Risk factors for maxillofacial injuries in a Brazilian emergency hospital sample. J Appl Oral Sci. 2010;18(1):23-9.
14. Okoje, Alonge, Oluteye, et al. Changing pattern of Pediatric Maxillofacial Injuries at the Accident and Emergency Department of the University Teaching Hospital, Ibadan-A Four Year experience.
15. Parsa T, Geibel J. Initial Evaluation and Management of Maxillofacial Injuries.
16. Eggensperger N, Smolka K, Scheidegger B, Zimmermann H, Iizuka T. A 3-year survey of assault-related maxillofacial fractures in central Switzerland. J Craniomaxillofac Surg. 2007;35(3):161-7.
17. Erol B, Tanrikulu R, Gorgun B. Maxillofacial fractures; Analysis of demographic distribution and treatment in 2901 patients 925 years experience. Craniomaxillofac. Surg. 2004;32(5):308-13.
18. Oison RA, Fonseca RJ, Zeitler DL, Osbon DB. Fractures of the mandible; review of 580 cases. J Oral Maxillofac Surg. 1982;40(1):23-8.

19. Lida S, Kogo M, Sugura T, Mima T, Matsuya T. Retrospective analysis of 1502 patients with facial fractures. Int J Oral Maxillofac Surg. 2001;30:256-90.
20. Lida S, Matsuya T. Pediatric maxillofacial fracture; their etiological characters and fracrure patterns. J Craniomaxillofac Surg. 2002;30:237-41.
21. Klenk G, Kovecs A. Etiology and patterns of facial fractures in the United Arab Emirates. J Craniomaxillofac Surg. 2003;14:78-84.
22. Gerbino G, Roccia F, Benech A, Caldarelli C. Analysis of 158 frontal sinus fractures: current surgical management and complications. J Craniomaxillofac Surg. 2000;28(30):133-9.
23. Lee KH, Snape L, Steenberg LJ, Worthington J. Comparision between interpersonal violence and motor vehicle accident in the etiology of maxillofacial fractures. ANZ J Surg. 2007;77:695-8.
24. Montovani JC, Campos LM, Moraes VM, Fereira FD, Nogueira EA. Etiology and incidence of facial fractures in children and adults (in Portuguese). Rev Bras Otorinolaryngol. 2006;72:235-41.
25. Qudah MA, Batanineh AB. A retrospective study of selected oral and maxillofacial ractures in a group of Jordanian children. Oral Surg Oral Med Oral Pathol Oral Radiol Endod. 2002;94:310-4.
26. Roccia F, Diasspro A, Nasi A, Berrone S. Management of sports related maxillofacial injuries. J Craniofac Surg. 2008;19(2):377-82.
27. Gassner P, TulI T, Hachi O, RUdisch A, Ulmer H. Craniomaxillofacial fractures–a 10-years revie of 9543 cases with 2106 injuries. Craniomaxillofac Surg. 2003;31(3):51-61.
28. Rosen P, Barkin R, Danzl F, et al. Emergency Medicine; Concepts and Clinical ractice, 4th edition. St Louis, Mosby Year book. 1998;p457.
29. Teasdale G, Jennett B. Assessment of coma impaired consciousness: LANCET. 1974;(ii):81-4.
30. Herbella FA, Mudo M, Delmonti C, Braga FM, Del Grande JC. 'Raccoon eyes' (periorbital haematoma) as a sign of skull base fracture. Injury. 2001;32(10):745-7.

CHAPTER

10 Idiopathic Sudden Sensorineural Hearing Loss

DEFINITION

Idiopathic sudden sensorineural hearing loss (SSNHL) has been defined as 30 dB or more sensorineural hearing loss over at least three contiguous audiometric frequencies, occurring within 3 days or less.

INCIDENCE

About 15,000 new cases are reported annually, worldwide.

Although the natural course of disease has not been established in a large number of patients, spontaneous recovery is variably reported to occur in up to 65% of patients who have idiopathic SSNHL. Much of the recovery is thought of as occurring within first month after the SHL.

Definition of "Improvement" or "recovery" is an improvement of 10 dB in pure tone average or an improvement of 10% or 15% in speech discrimination score (SDS). In most cases, an audiogram before SHL is not available and must be assumed.

ETIOLOGY

The etiology of SSNHL is idiopathic but viral infection, vascular compromise, disruption of cochlear membrane, immunological diseases and otologic tumors can cause hearing loss.

One third of patients have upper respiratory prodrome preceding SSNHL, suggesting the role of viruses in the etiology of this disease. The alteration in microcirculation of cochlear has been long suggested to be a cause. The blood supply to cochlea is by labyrinthine artery, which has no collateral vasculature. Vascular disorders may cause SSNHL because of cochlear injury and dysfunction secondary to anoxia or hypoxia.

List of potential etiologies is given in Table 10.1.

Table 10.1 Potential etiologies of SSNHL

Infectious causes	
Meningitis (streptococcal, meningococcal, cryptococcal)	Lassa fever
Mumps	HIV/AIDS
Rubeola	Mononucleosis
Rubella	Mycoplasma
Syphilis	Toxoplasmosis
Herpes virus (simplex, zoster, varicella)	Cytomegalovirus
Toxic causes	
Snake bite	Ototoxic agents
Immunological causes	
Wegener's granulomatosis	Primary immune inner ear diseases
Cogan's syndrome	
Other causes	
Hyperostosis cranialis interna	Pseudohypacusis
Neoplastic causes	
Acoustic neuroma	Leukemia
Meningioma	Myeloma
Lymphoma	Meningeal carcinomatosis
Neurological causes	
Multiple sclerosis	Neurosarcoidosis
Circulatory causes	
Cerebrovascular accident	Cardiopulmonary bypass
Sickle cell disease	Vertebrobasilar insufficiency
Traumatic causes	
Temporal bone fracture	Perilymph fistula
Acoustic trauma	Otologic surgery
Barotrauma	

EVALUATION

Goal is to detect known cause of SHL.

History Taking

The main elements include:

- Time of onset
- Progression of fluctuation since onset

- The presence or absence of neurological deficits
- Vestibular symptoms, tinnitus or aural fullness
- Aural pain
- Upper respiratory tract infection
- Trauma
- Autoimmune diseases in patient or family members
- Ototoxic agents.

Otolaryngological Examination

- Otoscopic examination to rule out infection, effusion, neoplasm
- Neurological examination including cranial nerve and cerebellar function
- Nasal septum—for evidence of autoimmune processes
- Tuning fork tests.

Audiometric Evaluation

- Pure tone audiogram and speech discrimination score to evaluate severity of initial loss and degree of recovery
- MRI of brain and internal auditory canals enhanced with gadolinium contrast
- CT scan with contrast, if MRI is contraindicated
- Laboratory evaluations including complete blood count, metabolic panels, electrolytes, erythrocyte sedimentation rate, rheumatological workup.

MANAGEMENT

Medical treatment should be started immediately after diagnosing, without any delay, if no identifiable cause is found. Treatment is not helpful after 30 days have passed because active disease may have resolved and damage may be permanent. The medical literature contains innumerable reports touting various treatment agents and regimens.

Combination of commonly employed regimens are:

- *Steroids:* They are mainstay of treatment of SSNHL as a result of high anti-inflammatory effect, they reduce cytotoxic immune response and increase microvascular blood flow in cochlea.

  Dosage: Intravenous methylprednisolone 1000 mg for 3 days combined with oral prednisolone taper, starting 60 mg daily, or intravenous hydrocortisone 100 mg twice daily for 2 days, this is followed by oral steroids in full therapeutic dose (either prednisolone 1 mg/kg or methylprednisolone 0.8 mg/kg) for 5 days. Dose is tapered over the next 10 days
- *Low molecular weight dextrans:* They cause expansion of plasma volume, increase in cardiac output, increase in vascular perfusion and microcirculation.

Dosage: Intravenous dextrans 5% dextrose in 500 mL, infused slowly over 4–6 hours, followed 2 hours later by another 500 mL, if patient has subjective improvement. Audiometry is repeated on second day. If patient has improvement another two units of 500 mL of 5% dextrose are infused over 6–8 hours. From third day, patient is treated with oral xanthinol nicotinate 150 mg, twice daily for 1 month. In diabetics, dextrans can be infused with normal saline instead of 5% dextrose

- Oral valacyclovir for viral infection being probable etiology
  Dosage: 500 mg three times daily for 10 days
- Neurovitamins B_1, B_2, B_3, B_6, B_{12}
- Aspirin 75 mg, twice daily to prevent thrombus formation
- Transtympanic steroids result in higher concentration of steroids in labyrinth. The main protocols for treatment in SSNHL is
  - Initial or primary treatment for SSNHL without systemic steroids
  - Adjunctive treatment given concomitantly with systemic steroids
  - "Salvage therapy" after failure of systemic steroids for SSNHL
- Hyperbaric oxygen
- Ginkgo biloba
- Dietary/lifestyle modification
  - Restriction of caffeine
  - Cessation of smoking.

BIBLIOGRAPHY

1. Anderson RG, Meyerhoff WL. Sudden sensory neural hearing loss. Otolaryngol Clin North Am. 1983;16:189-94.
2. Choung YH, Park K, Shin YR, Cho MJ. Intratympanic dexamethasone injection for refractory sudden sensory neural hearing loss. Larngoscope. 2009;116:747-52.
3. Hughes GB, Freeman MA, Haberkamp TJ, Guay ME. Sudden sensorineural hearing loss. Otolaryngol Clin North Am. 1996;29:393-405.
4. Mattox DE, Lyles CA. Idiopathic sudden sensorineural hearing loss. Am J Otol. 1989;10: 242-7.
5. Nan L, Wilson WR. Predictive recovery from idiopathic suddenhearing loss. Am J Otol. 1983;4:161-4.
6. O' Malley MR, Hayens DS. Sudden hearing loss. Otolaryngol Clin North Am. 2008;41(3): 633-9.
7. Vijayendra H, Buggaveeti G, Parikh B, Sangitha R. Sudden sensorineural hearing loss: An Otologic Emergency, Indian J Otolaryngol Head Neck Surg. 2012; 64(1):1-4.
8. Westerlaken BO, de Kleine E, Van der Laan B, Albers F. Treatment of sudden sensorineural hearing loss with pulse therapy: A prospective, randomized, double-blind clinical trial. Laryngoscope. 2007;117:684-90.
9. Zadeh MH, Storper IS, Spitzer JB. Diagnosis and treatment of sudden onset sensorineural hearing loss: A study of 51 patients. Otolaryngol Head Neck Surg. 2003;128:92-8.

CHAPTER

11 Quinsy

Quinsy is also called as peritonsillar abscess.

Peritonsillar abscess (PTA) is the most common deep infection of the head and neck region. It is an emergency situation causing severe odynophagia and needs immediate drainage (Figure 11.1).

DEFINITION

It is the collection of pus in the peritonsillar space, which lies between the capsule of the tonsil and the superior constrictor muscle.

Quinsy usually arises as a complication of an untreated or partially treated tonsillitis.

TYPES

- Anterior presentation: It is the commonest type. The abscess tends to point through the anterior pillar
- Posterior presentation: It pushes the tonsil forwards

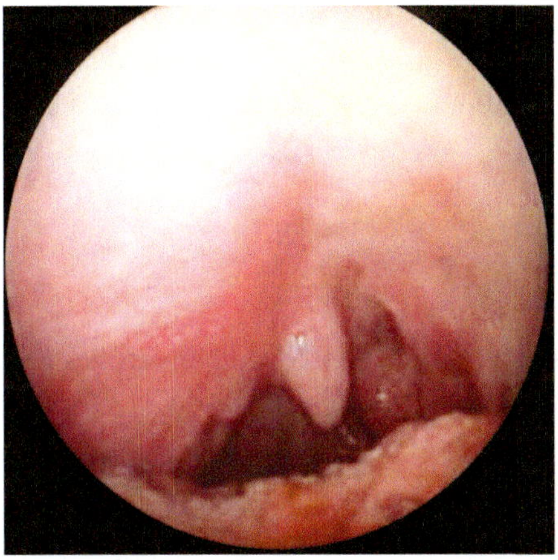

Figure 11.1 Peritonsillar abscess

- Lingual: The lower pole of the tonsil is affected
- Tonsillar: Quinsy is within the tonsil

ETIOLOGY

- Age: It occurs between the age of 20 to 50 years
- Sex: More common in males
- Recurrent tonsillitis acts as a predisposing factor
- Foreign body embedded in the substance of the tonsil may also lead to quinsy
- Tonsillar tag left behind after tonsillectomy may be affected by quinsy
- One of the important explanations for peritonsillar abscess is an abscess formation of Weber's salivary glands in the supratonsillar fossa
- Peritonsillar abscess can also occur de novo.

BACTERIOLOGY

Culture of pus from the abscess may reveal pure growth of *Streptococcus pyogenes*, *Staphylococcus aureus* or anaerobic organisms. More often the growth is mixed, with both aerobic and anaerobic organisms. It is most often caused by a type of bacteria called group-A β-hemolytic *Streptococcus*.

CLINICAL FEATURES

- It mostly affects adults and rarely the children, though acute tonsillitis is common among children
- Usually, it is unilateral.

Symptoms

General

- High fever
- Chills and rigors
- Malaise and body aches
- Dull headache
- Nausea and constipation.

Local

- Pain
  - Severe throat pain
  - Referred otalgia (via cranial nerve IX that supplies both the tonsils and the ear) in the ipsilateral side
  - Pain around the angle of mandible
- Odynophagia
  - Patient is unable to swallow even saliva, leading to drooling

- Trismus—due to spasm of masticator muscles, which are in close proximity with the superior constrictor
- Muffled and thick speech (distortion of vowels), often described as "Hot potato voice"
- Foul breath due to sepsis in the oral cavity and poor hygiene
- Restricted neck movements (Torticollis).

In typical cases, the patient puts his head forwards, bends the head slightly towards the affected side and has restricted neck movements.

Signs

- Tonsil is congested and bulged in one side
- Soft palate is edematous on the affected side
- Congestion and bulging of the soft palate, anterosuperior to the tonsil (Figure 11.2)
- Uvula is pushed to opposite side and edematous (Figure 11.3)

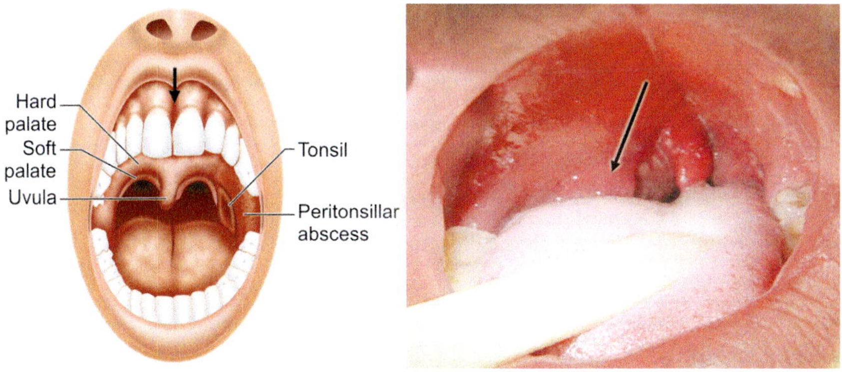

Figure 11.2 Bulging quinsy with deviated uvula

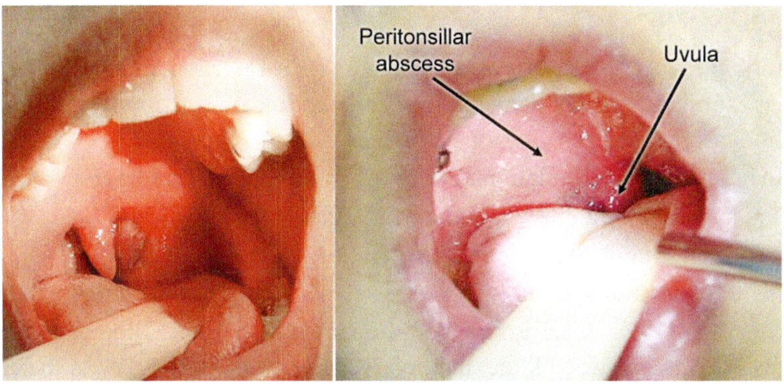

Figure 11.3 Peritonsillar abscess with edematous uvula

- Movement of palate is restricted
- Mucopus may be seen covering the tonsillar region
- Jugulodigastric node is enlarged and tender in the same side of quinsy.

DIFFERENTIAL DIAGNOSIS

- Acute tonsillitis—it is bilateral, pain is not severe and usually does not radiate to the ear
- Retropharyngeal abscess
- Parapharyngeal abscess
- Malignancy of the tonsil—lymphoepithelioma may mimic quinsy, but it is more chronic and less painful. It is hard to feel and pus does not drain on incising it.

COMPLICATIONS

- Parapharyngeal abscess
- Local venous thrombosis or phlebitis of the internal jugular vein may occur
- Septicemia may result from thrombophlebitis
- Hemorrhage may result from necrosis of internal carotid artery
- Supraglottic edema with obstruction to airway may occur.

  These days due to use of antibiotics, complications are rare.

DIAGNOSIS

- A thorough history and physical examination
- Ultrasonography
- CT scan (Figure 11.4)
- Needle aspiration (Gold standard) (Figure 11.5).

TREATMENT

Conservative

- Antibiotics: Antibiotics are also given to treat the infection. Internationally, the infection is frequently penicillin-resistant, so it is now common to treat with clindamycin[1]
- Analgesics and anti-inflammatory drugs to relieve pain and fever
- Oral hygiene maintained by antiseptic gargles
- Hydration should be maintained
- Incision and drainage.

Under 4% xylocaine, surface anesthesia with St. Clair Thompson quinsy forceps or with a guarded knife, incision is made on the soft palate at the site of maximum prominence. Incision is widened with long sinus forceps and purulent discharge is drained.

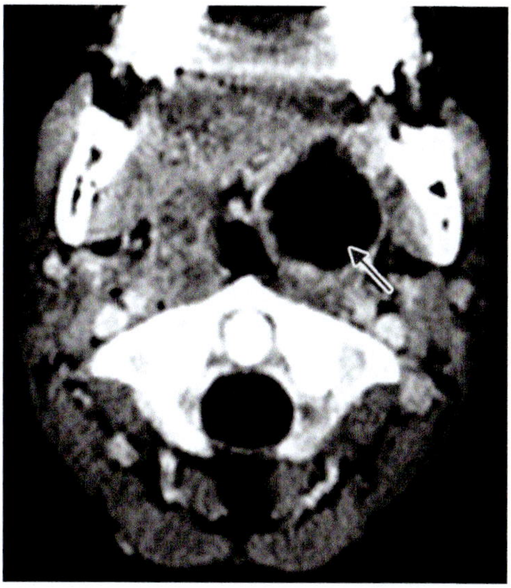

Figure 11.4 CT scan of quinsy

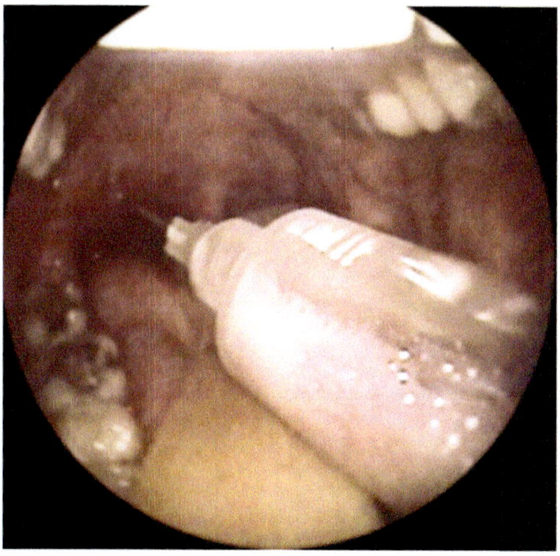

Figure 11.5 Needle aspiration

Site of Incision and Drainage (Figure 11.6)

- The most prominent site of the bulge
- A line drawn from the base of the uvula horizontally and a vertical line drawn from the anterior pillar intersect at a point near the superior pole. Incision is made superolateral to the intersection of these two lines
- Midway between upper last molar tooth and base of the uvula
- Through the intratonsillar crypt.

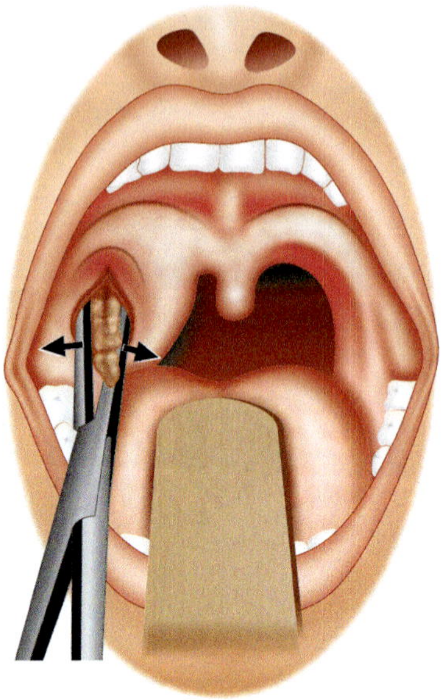

Figure 11.6 Site of drainage in quinsy

Tonsillectomy

After one attack of quinsy, the chance of recurrence is 20%. Therefore, a second quinsy is considered as an absolute indication for tonsillectomy, usually after an interval of 6 weeks.

Interval Tonsillectomy

In view of the painful nature of quinsy and its possible serious complications that may arise, tonsillectomy is advocated after 6 to 8 weeks, when inflammation has subsided.

Abscess Tonsillectomy or Hot Tonsillectomy or Quinsy Tonsillectomy

Some surgeons recommended it. Tonsillectomy is done at the same time as draining the abscess. It is done on the assumption that, since the tonsil forms the medial wall of the abscess, therefore, tonsillectomy gives drainage to the abscess as well as save the patient from interval tonsillectomy. However, this procedure is not favored as the abscess may rupture during anesthesia with consequent problems of aspiration. Besides, as the tissues are acutely inflamed, hence, there occurs severe bleeding and chances of systemic dissemination of infection are more. Chance of thromboembolism also there. The advantage of this is that, incision and drainage are avoided and only hospital admission is necessary.

Also, tonsillectomy is indicated in children who will not tolerate needle aspiration.

NOTABLE CASES

- Sultan Tekish of Kwarezm[3]
- George Washington was believed to have died of complications arising from quinsy, but is now thought to have died from epiglottitis[4]
- James Gregory of the band The Ordinary Boys almost died from quinsy because it was left untreated for so long before emergency treatment was started[5]
- Osceola[6]
- Michel de Montaigne.[7]

REFERENCES

1. Steyer TE. Peritonsillar abscess: diagnosis and treatment. Am Fam Physician. 2002;65 (1):93-6.
2. Greene RG. The International cyclopedia: a compendium of human knowledge. 1890;12:355-6.
3. Juvaini, Ala-ad-Din Ata-Malik. History of the World Conqueror. Manchester U.K.: Manchester University Press. 1997;314.
4. Plantation MV. Part 4. President and Back Home. Meet George Washington. Mount Vernon Ladies Association. 2006.
5. Ordinary Boys reveal illness that caused V cancellation. Retrieved 2006.
6. Wickman PR. Osceola's Legacy. University of Alabama Press. 2006;144.
7. de Michel M. Essays of Michel de Montaigne tr. 1877. In Charles Cotton (Ed). William Carew Hazlitt, 1877, The Life of Montaigne in v. 1. n.p., Kindle edition.

CHAPTER

12 Malignant Otitis Externa with Skull Base Osteomyelitis

INTRODUCTION

Skull base osteomyelitis (SBO) is one of the devastating infection with potential morbidity and mortality, which warrants a high degree of suspicion when formulating a differential diagnosis for otologic and skull base lesions. Malignant external otitis (MEO) is a more localized form of skull base osteomyelitis, which usually spreads to periauricular soft tissue, cartilage and bone. If untreated, it may extend throughout the skull base, infratemporal fossa, parapharyngeal space, nasopharynx and finally spreads intracranially. Other pathologies in this area with similar symptoms and signs are Wegener's granulomatosis, carcinoma of temporal bone, carcinoma of nasopharynx, metastatic lesion to clivus, Paget's disease, fibrous dysplasia and basilar skull fracture. Osseous skull base is made up of tympanic ring, mastoid, petrous, maxillary, ethmoid, sphenoid and occipital bones. Osteomyelitis of the skull base involves an infection in the diploic cancellous bone of the outer and/or inner cortical and periosteum, the dura, surrounding soft tissue, major vessels and cranial nerves of skull base.

The original report was by Melzter and Kelemen[21] in 1959, described as a case of *pyocyaneus*. Chandler[4] in 1968 was credited with coining the term malignant external otitis (MEO). The term malignant is used to emphasize the serious nature of this infection, as in the original historical report 7 of the 13 patients died. Various alternative terms used are (synonyms)—progressive, fulminant, invasive and necrotizing otitis externa (NOE).

Lucent et al.[17] described the term MEO as a dangerous misnomer. But despite these misgivings, the term MEO is widely used in the literature. NOE has been offered as an alternative term of MEO, which is a more limited form of infection, isolated to the skin and cartilage of the ectopic autologous cartilage (EAC), which may not always be associated with *Pseudomonas* infection, but may be with others like *Staphylococcus*.

ETIOPATHOLOGY

In a comprehensive review of literature on osteomyelitis, Waldrogel et al.[31] noted three fundamental factors for the pathogenesis—a contagious focus of infection, hematogenous seeding and microvascular diseases. Known microangiopathy of elderly diabetic, with poor glucose control, compromises blood supply to the affected area that limits effective immunological response and host resistance. The most common factor identified in the majority of the cases with MEO is the existence of elderly diabetes mellitus (90%) and majority are aged 60 years or older. Other predisposing factors are use of hearing aid, chronic suppurative otitis media (CSOM), leukemia, alcoholism, kernicterus, tuberculosis, swimmers, etc. Rubin et al[25] in a retrospective study, found that 61.5% of patients with MEO had unsterile tap water irrigation of their ear within 2 weeks of onset of symptoms, which is iatrogenic by physicians.

Some of the other organisms have been identified in MEO and SBO, in both adults and childrens are *Salmonella.*[28] *Mycobacterium tuberculosis,*[14] *Actoinomyces,*[30] *Aspergillus flavus,*[22] *Aspergillus fumigatus.*[5] But *Pseudomonas* is found in 99.2% of cases of MEO.[15] Other organisms involved are *Staphylococcus aureus*[15] and *epidermidis.*[2]

The pathogenesis of SBO as outlined by Nado et al.[24] begins in the epithelium of the EAC and extends into the retromandibular fossa through the fissure of Santorini into the parotid space or through the tympanomastoid suture. Facial palsy is typically due to soft tissue infection around the stylomastoid foramen.

Infection spreads to mastoid tip and jugular foramen with potential thrombosis of the sigmoid sinus and lower cranial nerve paresis. Transvenous thrombosis and sepsis may affect lateral sinus, superior and inferior petrosal sinus with progressive osteomyelitis advancing into the petrous apex, middle fossa, base of sphenoid and clivus of the posterior fossa, contralateral temporal bone and skull base. Posterior spread into the occipital bone elicits neural pain and potential compromise of the contents in the posterior cranial fossa. It may also spread anteriorly into the temporal fossa and facial bone.

DIAGNOSIS

The diagnosis of MEO is based on clinical and laboratory evidence along with heightened suspicion of the physician. But there is no absolute diagnostic criteria. However, Cohen and Friedman[6] proposed diagnostic criteria by developing obligatory and occasional categories. The major obligatory criteria include pain, exudate, edema, granulation tissue, microabscess, positive technetium-99 scan or the failure of local treatment after more than 1 week and the presence of *Pseudomonas aeruginosa*. The minor occasional criteria include positive CT scan, old age, cranial nerve palsy, diabetes mellitus or other debilitating conditions. In the absence of otological complaints and findings, SBO may be difficult to diagnose. Isolated case reports have been published that review SBO without any history of ear infection. The clinician must be aware of any prior history of MEO despite having received successful treatment, as the classic presentation in these cases is that, patient leaves the hospital completely asymptomatic only to return 4 to 7 weeks later with the onset of low grade fever, malaise and a unilateral unremitting headache that requires narcotic analgesic. It has also been reported that SBO can develop nearly one year after resolution of MEO.[1] MEO is not unique to elderly diabetic patients alone but few cases are reported in pediatric population also with *Pseudomonas aeruginosa*[13] and *Proteus mirabilis*[7] infection. Disorders other than diabetes mellitus (DM) associated with MEO in children are anemia, malnutrition, SJ syndrome, IG deficiency[8] and agranulocytosis. It is proposed that the medial location[12] of the bony cartilaginous junction in infants and children account for earlier compromise of facial nerve and mastoid.

STAGING AND IMAGING

The importance of staging for SBO is to alert the clinician that certain diagnostic tests are necessary to determine the presence and extent of the disease. Baseline CT and radionuclide scans will attempt to differentiate NEO from MEO and SBO. Gallium-67 scanning identifies inflammation if immunocompetent white cells are present and functioning. The technetium-99 bone scan reflects the increased osteoblastic activity, which is indicative of osteitis and osteomyelitis. A three level staging is proposed by Benecke.[3] Stage I or NOE is limited disease in the soft tissue without bone involvement whereas stage II describes MEO in which the disease is limited to the mastoid and is the earliest form of SBO with positive gallium and technetium scan. Finally, Stage III is extensive SBO with markedly positive gallium and technetium scan. Another staging system is proposed by Davis[9] based on clinical criteria and prognosis in three stages.

A third staging system was proposed by Krum, Rehm and Kenny,[16] which describe Stage-I: MEO limited to the EAC and mastoid air cells, Stage-II: SBO with cranial nerve palsy and Stage-III: Extension to the brain and meninges. Radiographic and radionuclide including Indium-III play an important role in evaluating, staging and managing MEO and SBO. Sequential imaging is critical in establishing diagnosis, demonstrating extent of the disease, monitoring the efficacy of treatment and determining the duration and end point of therapy.

TREATMENT

The complex management of MEO and SBO consists of—establishing the diagnosis, determining the extent of the disease, operating when indicated and providing appropriate antimicrobial therapy along with adjuvant therapy till the resolution of the infective process. It is also necessary to correct any metabolic abnormality and maintain glucose levels. The role of surgery is not very well-defined except taking biopsy and local debridement of necrotic tissue and drainage of abscess or formal tympanomastoid procedures like modified radial mastoidectomy (MRM) or radical mastoidectomy with partial petrous apicoectomy and embolectomy for jugular vein thrombosis. Farrier[10] proposed planned surgical debridement for persistent pain or failure of the granulation tissue to heal after 2 weeks of IV antibiotics. Raines and Schindler[26] advocated radical surgery on new onset of cranial neuropathies directly in recalcitrant MEO. Concern exists that surgery may enhance MEO and SBO by opening up facial spaces and new tissue plane with spreading infection. Prolonged antibiotic therapy with third generation cephalosporins has been the principal mean of therapy. Management of MEO and SBO significantly changed in the last decade with the availability of oral fluroquinolones like ciprofloxacin and ofloxacin.[29] In a report by Rubin et al.[27] patients were cured of MEO with the combination of ciprofloxacin and rifampicin for 6 to 12 weeks. Oral ciprofloxacin alone in 750 mg BID dose cured 21 out of 23 patients treated by Lang.[18] Ciprofloxacin given orally for a minimum of 6 weeks to 6 months was successful in patients who failed in conventional combination intravenous therapy. Similar efficacy with ofloxacin (200 mg) BD given to 17 patients with MEO achieved subjective improvement in all patients within 6 days and objective improvement within 12 days of treatment.[19,20] Despite the reported efficacy of prolonged systemic antibiotic therapy, treatment failure do occur due to tissue hypoperfusion and hypoxia, where the use of hyperbaric oxygen (HBO) increases wound PO_2 levels, enhances phagocytic oxidative killing of aerobic microorganisms, promotes angioneogenesis and osteoneogenesis. Treatment consists of 100% O_2 given for 90 minutes at 2.5 atm absolute pressure 5 days a week for 4 weeks as an adjuvant therapy.[23]

COMPLICATIONS AND PROGNOSIS

Cranial nerve neuropathy is the most common noniatrogenic complication in MEO and SBO. *Pseudomonas aeruginosa* produces destructive enzymes and exotoxins that promote tissue necrosis and reversible neurotoxicity.[32] Other than facial palsy, the jugular foramen syndrome affecting 9th, 10th and 11th cranial nerves compromising phonation, swallowing and protection of the tracheobronchial tree. Other cranial nerves, which may be affected are 3rd, 5th and 6th. In untreated or advanced cases, death results, due to meningitis, cerebritis, cerebral abscess, jugular foramen syndrome, pulmonary aspiration and pneumonia, vascular thrombosis, cerebrovascular accident (CVA) or subarachnoid hemorrhage. The mortality rate is high with multiple cranial neuropathies despite optimal antimicrobial therapy. However, recent reports with appropriate antibiotic therapy shows cure rates to be 80–100%. Use of hyperbaric O_2 as an adjuvant therapy has further reduced the mortality rate.

SUMMARY AND CONCLUSION

Skull base osteomyelitis is an aggressive, invasive, indolent infection with potentially significant morbidity and mortality. The most common form of SBO is MEO, typically seen in elderly diabetics although infections may be from other neurosurgical and cranial base sources or procedures. The diagnosis is based on detailed history, clinical evaluation, culture, biopsy, blood sugar, ESR and imaging studies. Intravenous antipseudomonal antibiotic therapy, surgical debridement of granulation tissue, bony sequestration and devitalized tissue from EAC can control and cure the disease effectively. Treatment for recalcitrant infections can be supplemented with adjuvant hyperbaric oxygen (HBO) therapy. The course of antibiotic therapy varies from a short 2 to 3 weeks for MEO in children to 6 months for SBO in adults. The duration of therapy is determined by number of factors including symptomatic and clinical response and demonstration of the resolution of inflammation by monitoring treatment with sequential CT, gallium scan and ESR. The overall morbidity and mortality have significantly declined with current methods of diagnosis and treatment during the past three decades when MEO was first described.

REFERENCES

1. Ame Dee, Mann WJ. Osteomyelitis of the skull base—an unusual manifestation. American Journal of Otolaryngology. 1989;10(5):402-4.
2. Brown HN, Levenson MJ. Necrotising MEO caused by *Staphylococcus epidermidis.* Arch ORL HNS. 1992;118:94-6.
3. Beneeke JE. Management of OSB Laryngoscope. 1989;99:1220-3.
4. Chandler JR. Malignant external Otitis: Laryngoscope. 1968;78:1257-94.
5. Cunningham M, et al. MEO due to *Aspergillus* in an immunocompetent patient. Arch ORSHNS. 1988;114:554-6.
6. Cohen D, Freidman P. The diagnostic criteria of MEO. J Laryngol Itol. 1987;101:216-21.
7. Coser Pl, et al. MEO in infants. Laryngoscope. 1980;90:312-6.
8. Castro R, et al. MEO and mastoiditis associated with an IgG4 subclass, deficiency in an child. Del Med J. 1990;62(12):1417-21.
9. Davis JC, et al. Adjuvant hyperbaric O_2 in MEO. Arch ORS HNS. 1992;118:89-93.
10. Farrior J. Osteomyelitis of the skull base. South Med J. 1989;82:719-22.
11. Grabman IR, et al. A typical osteomyelitis of skullbase. Laryngoscope. 1989;99:671-6.
12. Horn KL and Gherinis. MEO of childhood. Amer J Otol.1981;2(4):402-4.
13. Jochims Hz. MEO in children. Arch Otolaryngol. 1985;111:406-8;1979;102:236-7.
14. Kearns DB, et al. Tuberous petrous apicitis. Arch Otolaryngol. 1985;111:406-8.
15. Keay DG, Muray JAM: MEO due to *Staphylococcus* infection. J Laryngol Otol. 1988;102:926-7.
16. Krans DH, Rehm SJ, Kineey SE. The evolving treatment of NEO. Laryngoscope. 1988;9: 934-9.
17. Lucente FE, et al. Malignant otitis externa: a dangerous misnomer. J ORL HNS. 1982;90:266-9.
18. Laug R, et al. Successful treatment of MEO with oral ciprofloxacin report of experience with 23 patients. J Infect Dis. 1990,161:537-40.
19. Levenson HJ, et al. Ciprofloxacin: drugs of choice in the treatment of MEO. Laryngoscope. 1991;101:821-4.

20. Levy R, et al. Oral Ciprofloxacin as treatment of MEO. A study of 17 cases. Laryngoscope. 1990;1000:548-51.
21. Meltzer PE, Kelemen G. Pyocynaneous Osteomyelitis of the temporal bone, Mandible and Zygoma.
22. Menachof MR, Jackler RK. Otogenic skull base Osteomyelitis caused by invasive fungal infection. ORLHNS. 1990;102:285-9.
23. Mader JT, Lone JT. MEO cure with HBO as adjuvant therapy Arch, ORL. 1982;108:38-40.
24. Nadol JB. Histopathology of *Pseudomonas* Osteomyelitis of the temporal bone starting as MEO. Amer J Oto Laryngol. 1980;1(5):359-71.
25. Rubin J. et al. Aural irrigation with water, a potential pathogenic mechanism for inducing MEO, Ann Otol Rhinolaryngol. 1990;99:117-9.
26. Raines J, Schindler RA. The surgical management of recalcitrant MEO. Laryngoscope. 1980;90:369-378.
27. Rubin J, et al. Efficacy of oral ciprofloxacin plus rifampicin for treatment of MEO. Arch ORL HNS. 1989;113:1063-9.
28. Senegor M, Levis HP. Salmonella Osteomyelitis of skullbase. Surg Neurol. 1991;36:37-39.
29. Strauss M. Current therapy of MEO, DRL HNS. 1990;102:174-6.
30. Vannior JP, etal. Actinomycotic Osteomyelitis of the skull base and altas with late dissemination. A case of transient neurological syndrome. Eur J Pediatrics. 1986;145(4):316-8.
31. Waldrogel FA, et al. Osteomyelitis: A review of clinical features therapeutic consideration and unusual aspects. N Engl J Med. 1970;282:198-206.
32. Lee WC, JF Sharp. Bing-neel syndrome or MEO in Waldenstrom's macroglobinemia. J laryngol and Otol. 1994;108:492-3.

CHAPTER

13 Foreign Body Airway Obstruction

The clinical problem presented by aspiration of foreign objects into the air passage ranges from the urgent fatal lodgement in the larynx to more subtle symptomatology where the object may get lodged in the peripheral bronchus.

Patients who are in imminent danger of death may require emergency tracheostomy.

ETIOLOGY

The tendency of small children to put whatever comes into their grasp into their mouths is well known. To this hasty eating and drinking, permitting children to play while eating, talking with food in mouth, giving peanuts to children who do not have proper molar teeth to chew them, improper supervision of children in the vicinity of infants who thrust foreign body into the younger ones.

PREDISPOSING FACTORS

- Age: Children less than 5 years of age constitute more than 50% of the patients. They have a tendency to put the things in their mouth, which can go either in the food or the air passages
- Cranial nerve IX (glossopharyngeal) and X (vagus) lesions: Paralysis of pharynx causes aspiration problems.

INCIDENCE

Foreign body removal accounts for about 5% of all pediatric endoscopic procedures; half of which are contributed by foreign body in the bronchus.

NATURE OF FOREIGN BODIES

- *Non-irritating:* Plastic, glass or metallic items may remain symptomless for a long time

- *Irritating:* Vegetables (peanuts, beans, seeds) can cause diffuse reactive congestion and edema of the tracheobronchial mucosa (vegetable bronchitis). They may swell up, and cause airway obstruction and pulmonary suppuration.

HISTORY

Often the child presents after a sudden episode of coughing, chocking while eating with subsequent wheezing, coughing, or stridor. However, in many cases chocking episode is not recalled at the time of history taking as the event would have occurred more than a week or even month before presentation.

CLINICAL FEATURES

Children may either hide or forget the incidence of foreign body (FB) inhalation. It is the suspicion of clinician that helps in diagnosis. Patients having FB in the air passage can pass through three stages:

- *Inhalation:* This is the initial period of choking, gagging and wheezing that lasts for a short time. Small FB may be coughed out. If it is large, patient may get cyanosis and die
- *Latent:* During this symptom free interval, mucosa adapts to the presence of FB. It varies with the size and nature of the FB. Nonvegetable FB may go unnoticed for a long period of time
- *Manifestation:* Depending on the site, size, shape and nature of the FB, the obstruction, inflammation and trauma to the airway can give rise to following features:
  - *Laryngeal foreign body:* A large FB can kill the person. A relatively small FB can present with throat discomfort, hoarseness of voice, croupy cough, aphonia, inspiratory stridor, dyspnea, and hemoptysis
  - *Tracheal foreign body:* A Sharp FB produces coughing and hemoptysis. A small seed may move up and down the trachea, and produce audible slap, tracheal flutter, and palpatory thud. Biphasic stridor or asthmatoid wheeze is best heard when child's mouth is open
  - *Bronchial foreign body:* Right bronchus is the most common site for lodgement for FBs as it is wider and more in line with lumen of tracheal lumen. A FB may either totally obstruct a lobar/segmental bronchus (atelectasis), or produce a check valve obstruction (obstructive emphysema) which allows only ingress.

DIFFERENTIAL DIAGNOSIS FOR RESPIRATORY DISTRESS

- Obstruction by foreign body
- Iatrogenic
  - Laryngeal nerve paralysis

- Tracheal ulceration or granuloma
- Vocal cord granuloma
- Infections
  - Croup/Epiglottitis
  - Diphtheria
  - Retropharyngeal or peritonsillar abscess
  - Pneumonia
- Neoplasms
  - Hemangiomas
  - Lymphangiomas
  - Recurrent respiratory papillomatosis
- Others
  - Asthma
  - Bronchitis
  - Lingual thyroid
  - Congenital craniofacial anomalies
  - Allergic edema.

WORK UP: IMAGING

Radiography

Most aspirated foreign bodies are food material and are radiolucent. Thus, one has to look indirectly for signs of the foreign body.

If the diagnosis is in doubt, pediatric radiologists can be helpful if they know the child is being evaluated for a foreign body.

A plain radiograph can reveal an area of focal over inflation or an area of atelectasis, depending on the degree of obstruction.

Aspirated foreign body lodged in the right main stem bronchus leading to hyperinflation (Figure 13.1A).

If the material completely occludes the left main stem bronchus, the radiograph may reveal opacification of the distal lung as residual air is absorbed and no air entry is possible (Figure 13.1B).

If the plain radiography findings are not diagnostic, remember that an affected lung portion does not completely empty. If the child cooperates, an anteroposterior expiratory radiograph may reveal trapped air in the affected portion of the lung. In those children who cannot cooperate with the maneuver, lateral decubitus radiographs may reveal the trapped air. An anteroposterior film with compression on the abdomen, mimicking a forced exhalation, can be helpful.

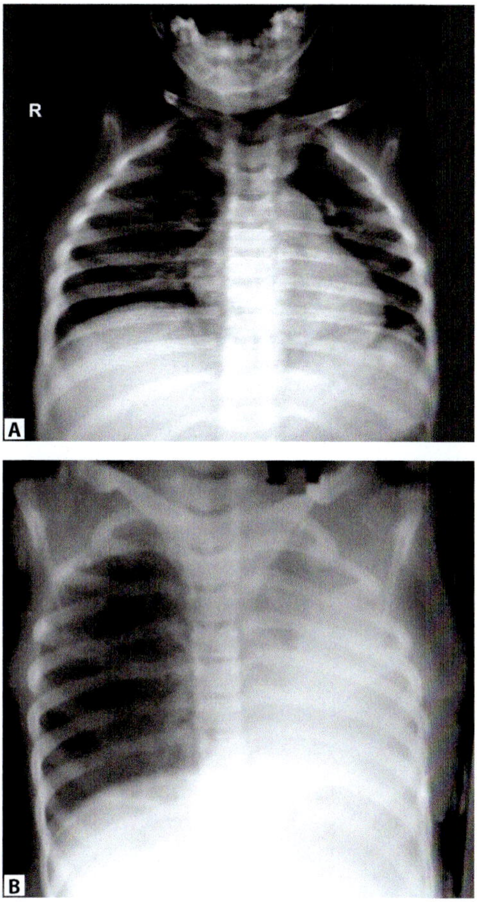

Figures 13.1A and B (A) Foreign body in right main bronchus leading to hyperinflation; (B) Foreign body in left main bronchus

Fluoroscopy

Fluoroscopy of the chest may be helpful in showing focal air trapping, paradoxical diaphragmatic motion, or both.

CT Scanning

Chest CT scanning may reveal the material in the airway, focal airway edema, or focal over-inflation not detected using plain radiography. If the index of suspicion is high, many physicians forgo CT scanning and proceed to the more definitive study, bronchoscopy.

Even if no foreign body is evident on any of the radiographic studies, a foreign body may still be present, and a bronchoscopy should be performed if the suspicion is high.

Management

- Medical: Antibiotics, steroids and oxygen are administered immediately, and continued after the bronchoscopy
- Laryngeal foreign body:
  - Cricothyrotomy or emergency tracheostomy: These are done when Heimlich's maneuver fails
  - Direct laryngoscopy or by laryngofissure: FB is removed by direct laryngoscope or by laryngofissure
- Heimlich's maneuver:
  - Indication: A large bolus of food completely obstructing the larynx with total aphonia, and patient dying of asphyxia (impending death)
  - Contraindication: Partially obstructing FB, because maneuver can cause total obstruction
  - Method: First pound on the back, and turn the patient upside down. Then, follows Heimlich maneuver. Stand behind the patient, and place arms around patient's lower chest giving four abdominal thrusts. The residual pulmonary air can dislodge the laryngeal FB.
- Tracheal and bronchial foreign bodies

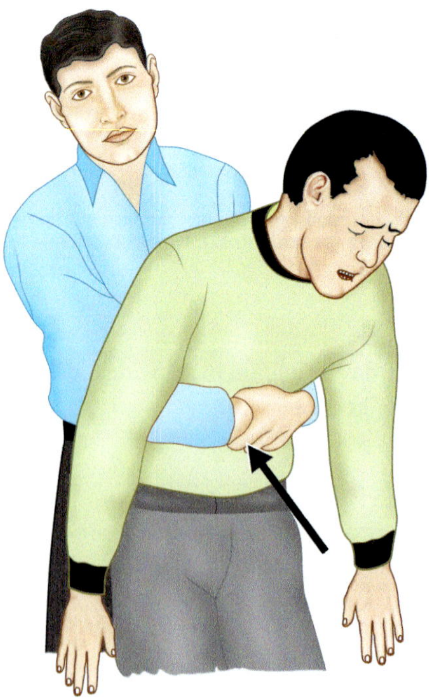

Figure 13.2 Heimlich's maneuver

- Bronchoscopy under general anesthesia: Rigid bronchoscopy is the standard procedure for FB removal. Emergency removal is indicated only when the airway obstruction is present or FB is vegetable. The following methods are used for the removal of tracheobronchial FB. Tracheal foreign body should be pushed to the either bronchus before retrieval as it is difficult to grasp FB:
  - Rigid bronchoscopy with or without a telescope
  - Bronchoscopy with C-arm fluoroscopy
  - Snares and basket of Fogarty's catheter balloon for rounded FB
  - Bronchoscopy through the tracheostome
  - Flexible fiberoptic bronchoscopy in selected cases
  - Thoracotomy and bronchotomy for peripheral foreign bodies
  - Lobectomy or pneumonectomy may be needed in cases of old unnoticed FB's.

PROCEDURE

Technique of Bronchoscopy

After selecting an appropriate size bronchoscope according to the age of the child, it should be checked for proper illumination and cleaned thoroughly. A correct size suction cannula should be checked and passed through the bronchoscope. Out of various types of FB forceps like toothed, non-toothed, cupped, serrated, flat, crocodile, alligator, etc. selection should be done keeping in mind the type of bronchial FB which can assure a firm grip of the FB without damaging the bronchial mucosa. After visualizing the larynx, after lifting the epiglottis by the laryngoscope, the bronchoscope should be gently introduced into the glottis with the tip upwards and under the epiglottis. Bronchoscope should be held in the right hand with penhold grip and should be gently slided into the trachea after visualizing the vocal chords. The anesthetist should then start inflating the lungs with Jet ventilation by the side of the bronchoscope. Failure to inflate the lungs with Jet ventilation and inability to identify the tracheal rings should alert that the bronchoscope is not in the air passage but in the esophagus. After it is confirmed that the endoscope is in trachea then it should be glided down over the left hand fingers without undue force and always under vision. The next step is the identification of cornea and introduction of the bronchoscope into the right main bronchus with slight angulation towards the left. Then it can be withdrawn slightly and angled towards the right to visualize the left main bronchus. During the whole procedure, suction should be done from time to time to cleanse the secretions. The bronchus, bronchoscope and the FB should lie in one straight line before it is removed. The blades of FB forceps should be opened after it crosses the tip of the endoscope and then the FB should be caught firmly and brought near the tip of the bronchoscope. Then the bronchoscope alongwith the FB forceps should be gently withdrawn simultaneously till it reaches the glottis. After this, the bronchoscope should be tilted slightly upwards with the held FB to pass out through the posterior part of the glottis which is wider. Loose FB in trachea are more difficult which should not be caught directly when they are in the trachea, rather it should be pushed down to let them lodge in either main bronchus, usually the right main bronchus, after which it is easy to catch and remove. Otherwise, loose trachea FB may get stuck in the subglottis region which is the narrowest area in the airway, causing total airway obstruction until and unless removed as early as possible.

After the removal of the FB the anesthetist should oxygenate the child and allow the endoscopist to reintroduce the bronchoscope for inspection of tracheobronchial tree for any remnant of FB or a second FB rarely. The tracheobronchial tree should be cleaned with suction and bronchoscope should be kept in trachea for proper oxygenation till the breathing is spontaneous. Both the surgeon and anesthetist should observe the child till the muscle tone returns to normal, cough reflex is present and child starts crying and air entry is checked on either side. The child should be kept in left lateral position before shifting to ward and if there is any evidence of subglottis edema in the form of brassy cough or stridor, then IV steroid should be given including strict observation of child.

BIBLIOGRAPHY

1. Evans JNG. Foreign bodies in the larynx and trachea, Scott Brown's diseases of Ear, Nose & Throat. 1997;6:1-11.
2. Rajasekaran S, BalaChandran K, Anbalagan S, Satish Kumar P, Vikram VJ. Management of Tracheobronchial Foreign Bodies in Children—A Retrospective study of series of 50 cases. Otolaryngology. 2013;3(3):3.
3. Rothman BF, Braeckman CR. Foreign bodies in larynx and tracheo bronchial tree in children. Review of 225 cases. Ann Oto Rhino laryngol. 1980;89:434-6.
4. Singh JK, Vasudevan V, Bharadwaj N, Narasimhan KL, Role of tracheostomy in the management of foreign body airway obstruction in children, Singapore Med J. 2009; 50(9):871-4.
5. Srppnath J, Mahendrakar V. Management of trachea bronchial foreign bodies—A retrospective analysis, Indian Journal of Otolaryngology and Head and Neck Surgery. 2002;54(2):127-131.

Index

Page numbers followed by *f* refer to figure and *t* refer to table

B

C

F

G

H

Q

R

S